Words of Life
for the Health of Soul and Body

*The eternal Word,
the One God, the Free Spirit,
speaks through Gabriele,
as through all the prophets of God —
Abraham, Job, Moses, Elijah, Isaiah,
Jesus of Nazareth,
the Christ of God*

Words of Life
for the Health
of Soul and Body

*This book is based on the
revelation of the Christ of God
"Cause and Development of All Illness"
Given through the teaching prophetess and
Emissary of God, Gabriele,
in the year 1986*

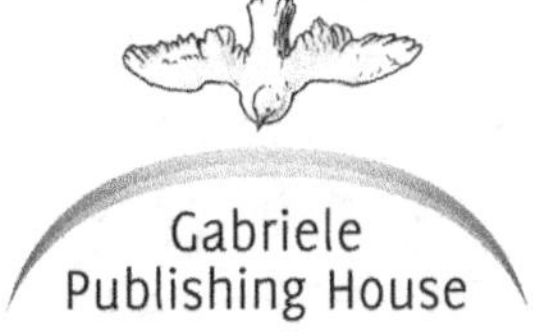

Gabriele
Publishing House

In Accompaniment

*It is not the reading of this book
that leads to health,
but the actualization of what
is recognized from it.*

*It is not the person's ego that heals,
but the I Am, the Spirit of Christ.*

*It is not self-love that makes us free,
but selfless love for God and for
all people and all Being.*

*Health, happiness, and freedom
are in ourselves.*

*This revelation of the Lord
shows us the way there.*

God, helps, relieves, and heals.

Gabriele

Table of Contents

Christ, the Lord, the Redeemer of human-kind, gave this fundamental revelation through Gabriele, the prophetess of God, in the mighty turn of time in which we find ourselves, It was in 1986—a time when on this Earth nature was still healthy to the extent that indications were given regarding the effects of natural remedies, water and sunlight that promote health.

In many revelations, which were partly given to humankind over 40 years ago—and particularly in this revelation "Cause and Development of All Illness"—the Spirit of the Christ of God repeatedly gave ever more urgent warning of the dangers threatening the world if humankind did not turn back and change its ways. If taken in time, a completely new orientation, through a spiritual orientation of the people in their way of thinking and living and through the fulfill-ment of the divine commandments, would have raised the vibration of the planet Earth. Humankind would have come into harmony with the high powers of life, which also maintain our planet and everything in and on it and lead to evolution.

God did not want destruction, suffering, hardship and horror for the Earth and for each of His human children, but evolution. But humankind did not pay attention to His admonishments and indications.

Meanwhile, what the Lord—also in this revelation—had warned us about years ago has come to pass. Nature is irreparably destroyed; a steadily increasing number of natural disasters announce the worse; the world and humankind are standing before the collapse. Because of the contamination of the Earth, the indications given by Christ, which refer to taking in the healing and life forces of nature, can no longer be applied in this way. The Earth can no longer produce the nutrients that it still could when this Christ-revelation was given.

What can the food of the future be like?—People's own gardens will again gain in significance!

But the world of materialism and of egocentric striving will pass away—it is thus revealed, and it will thus happen. A worldwide radical change such as has never been experienced before is in the offing. From the ashes of the human ego and from the floods of negative energy, which human beings created by disregarding the commandments of God, a spiritually oriented age is rising, a new humanity, which fulfills the commandments of heaven. After chaos and destruction, which are the effects of the causes created by humankind over thousands of years, the Kingdom of Peace of Jesus Christ will spread worldwide on the cleansed Earth.

What has been built up in the Spirit of God, in the following of the Nazarene and in fulfillment of the laws of God, that is, what emerged in God's will, will also be significant in the coming era of light. This also applies to this great Christ-revelation from the year 1986.

On the new, light-filled Earth, it will again be as it was originally. Nature will be healthy as will the nature bodies, the human beings. Then the fullness will be manifest, with which God cares for us, His children in the earthly garment—by way of nature. This book will then be a historical work.

Gabriele-Verlag Das Wort

Preface

Greetings in God, dear brothers, and sisters!

In the Spirit of the Lord all are brothers and sisters. Since I am giving a revelation from the Spirit of the Lord, I call all human beings my brothers and sisters, no matter their convictions.

My name is Brother Emanuel—this is how I am called on Earth in the work of the Lord, in Universal Life. My entity is a guardian of the law before the throne of God, the Cherub of divine Wisdom.

The following revelation, "Cause and Development of All Illness," is the word of Christ given to all humankind. His word flows through His instrument, whom He calls His prophetess. The word of God is the I Am, for God, the life, the I Am, is everything in all things.

The revelation of the Lord gives insight into the event of the Fall and deep knowledge from the law of sowing and reaping, the causal law. The eternal law as well as the causal law reflect the justice of God. Since everything is radiation, both laws, the eternal law and the causal law, are also based on cosmic radiation. Therefore, words can never express what the subtlest radiation reflects. Words are symbols or terms. Those who want to attain deeper insight into the words, who want to grasp their meaning, must decipher the words, which are only symbols and terms, and come to understand them according to their meaning.

Christ, the Redeemer of all human beings and souls, explains in His revelation "Cause and Development of All Illness" how, and in what way, the human being has created and still creates causes, how the causes became and become effective, what has resulted from them and what threatens to result from them in due course.

Christ, who inspired this revelation, "Cause and Development of All Illness," repeats essential knowledge several times, shedding light on His explanations again and again from different perspectives so that the reader can grasp the meaning—for manifold are the causes and effects that lead to worry, need, illness and suffering. May everyone show understanding for these repetitions. At first reading, every person grasps one principle of the law. If, however, it is examined from different sides and repeated several times, it can penetrate more deeply into the reader, and be grasped and actualized in its depths.

This revelation is meant to stimulate thought in all of humankind and to motivate the individuals to live their life earnestly—both in thought and word, as well as in the deed.

May many brothers and sisters awaken to knowledge and actualize the laws so that there may be light in this world!

Peace to all people and beings!
Brother Emanuel,
the Cherub of divine Wisdom.

God created the heavens and this Earth

God is the Spirit in Me, the Christ, the Redeemer of humankind, who is the word, this revelation.

The pure heavens, the heavenly beings and the spiritual nature kingdoms came into being through the Spirit of the eternal Father.

God created the heavens. The Earth and all part or fully material suns and worlds emerged from the Fall.

The condensed forms are condensed spirit.

Out of love for His fallen children, God allowed the condensation of the pure spirit—to grant His renegade children housing, food and everything needed for the human body—the housing of the soul. Therefore, it is said: God created the heavens and this Earth.

The spirit body, which is called "soul" in its burdened form, comes from the eternal heavens, the law, God. It has all the spiritual substances of infinity and is, therefore, a microcosm in the macrocosm, a being from eternity. Because of this, it is from eternity to eternity—that is, immortal.

The physical body, the human being—the soul's housing—is from the Earth and has only the substances of this Earth. For this reason, the body is capable of life only to a limited extent, as is the Earth itself. Matter consists of coarse matter and is relative and transitory in its forms.

The physical body, the coarse-material garment, the human being, the housing of the soul, is capable of life only through the eternal Spirit, God. The Spirit, God, is the life in all fine and coarse material forms of Being.

Without the Spirit, God, the life, no form can exist. Life reveals itself in manifold forms, both in the beings of heaven as in souls and human beings, in the mineral, plant and animal kingdoms.

All life is the revelation of God.

The Spirit, God, is also called the primordial energy because God is infinitely eternal. His workings are boundless. The Spirit, God, is omnipresent—unfathomable and eternally creative.

*The pure spiritual beings and forms
are an expression of the eternal Spirit—
the material ones are maintained by Him*

The Creator-Spirit, God, the primordial energy, brought and brings forth the spiritual forms, which are also called the pure forms of Being.

The heavens with their pure beings and spiritual forms are the expression of the Eternal. All material forms are maintained by the eternal Spirit, the divine ether stream.

All spiritual forms have the fully developed core of being or germ of being. Both are "switching points" for the inflowing divine stream, the divine energy, also called the ether stream.

In the heavenly minerals, plants and animals, the germ of being is only partly unfolded;

it evolves into the perfect core of being, which is fully developed and active in the pure spirit beings.

Thus, in its spiritual form, the pure spirit being is the Absolute Law itself.

The soul is also a pure spiritual structure but enveloped by garments that reflect the burdens that have been absorbed by the particles of the spirit body. Once the soul has discarded its garments, the coverings, its burdens, it has again become a pure spirit being, the compressed eternal law. It then returns to the Father-house. In the incarnated state, the spirit body is also called soul.

Therefore, the human being consists of a threefold unity—the spirit, also called primordial energy, the soul, and the coarse-material body. This threefold unity is called the human being.

The spirit body in its burdened condition is surrounded by seven basic ethereal garments. They reflect the burdens of the soul and characterize and mark the human being. Since every basic garment is reflected in every other garment, the result is seven times seven spectra of the soul. Every burden has its color and its sound in the orchestra of the satanic.

Therefore, the burdens, with their colors and sounds, mark and characterize the physical body. In this way, human beings are the expression, the radiation, of the soul. They are sound and melody according to their state of consciousness, their burden.

Like everything in infinity, the pure Being, the eternal heavens, consists of spiritual atoms. Matter consists of material atoms and molecules. All Being—the purely spiritual, as well as the part-material, the material, and the spheres of purification—is respirated by the eternal Spirit, the primordial energy, by way of the nucleus of the spiritual and material atoms. This means that they are supplied with life force. And in this way, all forms of life are held together.

The former spirit being, clothed as a soul in the garment, "human being," first of all, transformed down its earlier fine ethereal vibrations by its desire to be like God. In the gradual process of its encasement and condensation, which resulted in the human being, the enveloped spirit being, and later the human being, transformed the divine forces down more and more by continuously feeling, thinking, speaking, and acting unlawfully. The finest ether streams became ever coarser, and finally became coarse-material substance, matter. In this way, over billions upon billions of years, matter came into being.

When the Eternal, also called the All-Spirit, brought the All to life and created the pure spiritual suns, worlds and spirit beings, He gave His heritage as essence to the spirit beings, His children. This means that every spirit being of the heavens is the law and therefore, bears infinity in itself as essence, in its spiritual atomic structure.

Through this, the spirit beings remain in the unity consciousness, in God. They sense and act out of the law, God. What they sense is God's primordial sensation. What they accomplish is God's deed.

In this way, they are constantly one with God. God lives through them, and they live the law, God. Through this, they are images of the Father, an expression of God.

Like attracts like—Unlike repels unlike:
The Fall-beings separated from
the unity consciousness. Parts of the
spiritual planets were blasted off

Through the Fall-event, many spirit beings separated from the unity consciousness because they wanted to be like God Himself: omnipresent Spirit.

The Fall-event had far greater dimensions and effects than the first Fall-children could imagine:

Through the rebellious spirit beings, which created dissonances and contaminated themselves with these, parts of the spiritual planets on which these spirit beings and Fall-beings had their heavenly dwellings were affected, that is, contaminated. Parts of the heavenly bodies changed their frequencies and began to reel about. Through the turbulences, these parts of the spiritual planets were split off and flung into the universe where they then formed themselves in zones of lesser light.

The eternal law applies to heaven as well as to Earth. Those who separate from the All-unity, from the primordial life, which is love, will fall into states of turbulence, into a disharmonious rhythm, and will be unable to stay connected to the divine rhythm, to the All-harmony.

The spirit beings who had rebelled against the primordial principle—and had now become Fall-beings—could no longer be maintained by the harmoniously balanced part of the spiritual planet that had remained permeated with the radiation of the eternal law. Since the Fall-beings enveloped themselves with their own unlawful sensations, they were no longer attracted by the lawful parts of the spiritual planets. The eternal law is: Like attracts like, unlike repels unlike.

Through the will of God, represented by a prince of the law, the Fall-beings were then escorted out of the pure heavens to where the split-off parts of the planet had meanwhile formed themselves. These parts of the planet then attracted those spirit beings that corresponded to their frequencies. The subsequent changes of light that resulted in a further condensation and a yet deeper fall led to the planes of preparation, the part-material worlds, the spheres of purification and full matter.

God is love and pure life.

Pure creation creation is spiritual energy that has taken on form.

The pure spiritual forms—the spirit beings, animals, plants, minerals, suns, and worlds of the heavens—are pure fine-material structures, permeated by the primordial light via the prism suns, which are an expression of the natures and attributes of God. They are embedded in the all-pervading eternal stream, in the law, the Spirit, God.

This is why there are no shadows in the pure Being. Everything is light. All pure forms are likewise self-luminous. This happens as follows:

In every spiritual atom there is a switching point, a "germ of being," through which the All-power, the Spirit of God, flows into the spiritual forms. This switching point, the "germ of being," slowly develops into the "core of being."

The "germ of being" corresponds to the respective state of development of a spiritual form. The "core of being" is a perfect switching point. It exists only in the spiritual atoms of the pure spirit beings. All other switching points, that is, all "germs of being," reflect the flowing energy, God, to the same extent as the spiritual form has developed. By way of the switching point—the "germ of being" or the "core of being" in the spiritual atoms—every form begins to be self-luminous, according to its development.

The Primordial Central Sun, the majestic heavenly body of the eternal Father, shines into the germ of being of the spiritual atoms in the heavenly mineral, plant and animal realms or into the core of being of the spirit beings, by way of the suns of the natures and attributes, which are also called prism suns or secondary primordial suns. The germ of being and core of being then started to become active and radiate whatever is developed within them: The germ of being radiates the respective state of development of the form; the core of being radiates the mentality of the spirit being.

Every radiation is also color and sound.

All told, it is the pure symphony, God, which is also called the divine orchestra or the heavenly music of the spheres.

Since everything shines from within to without, there are no shadows.

All unlawfulness, all baseness, has to develop back to the All-harmony, God

The realms of the Fall, which are the planes of preparation and the planes of purification for disembodied souls and for matter, emerged through the Fall-event, because parts of the spiritual planets changed in rhythm and sound through the wrongdoing of the spirit beings. The further envelopment and condensation of these part-planets resulted from ever greater transgressions of the law by the spirit beings in their feeling, thinking and acting. The shells, the condensations of these part-planets, are thoughts that took on form.

All unlawfulness, all baseness, has to develop back to the highest and pure, from the thought vibration of the ego toward the All-harmony, God. The evolution of the soul back to God, the All-harmony, is accomplished through Me, Christ, the Redeemer of all human beings and souls. The transformation of the part-planets takes place through the primordial power, through the "Let there be."

In this revelation, I give you an overview of how the Fall came to pass and how the first causes were created, which then drew after themselves further causes and effects; for through this, suffering, hardship and illness emerged.

At the same time, however, I give insight into the eternal laws of My Father and show, often with repetitions, how human beings can avoid causes or clear them up in time, before they come into effect. I show how effects may be alleviated or eliminated through the behavior of the individual.

I will now start with a short explanation of how it came to the first Fall-thought—the desire to be like God.

Before the Spirit, God, gave life to infinity with spiritual forms of light, with spiritual stars and planets and with spiritual beings, animals, plants and minerals, His holy primordial light, the Spirit, shone in infinity. As long as these spiritual energies, the heavenly planets, spirit beings, animals, plants and minerals, had not yet taken on form and been brought into existence, the primordial energy, the light, God, was almost motionless. It shone.

In a cycle determined by the primordial energy itself, the primordial light, the primordial energy, began to move more intensely. Motion implies that something wants to take place. The primordial light became more active in its creative predispositions, the four natures of God. The primordial light now wanted to give itself form.

The active part of the creative energy had a stronger effect on the less active energy. Through this, what gradually emerged was an increasing interaction which produced further energies.

From the existing spiritual atoms, further spiritual atoms developed. In this way, the energy increased.

This means that at first, the four natures of God became more active; these then stimulated the three attributes of God to higher activity.

Once the seven basic powers were active, the primordial substance undertook a shifting of the energy. Until then, it had consisted of half positive and half negative forces. The shifting led to the formation of two-thirds positive and one-third negative forces. The result of this was the

Father-Mother-Principle, and thus, the creative and maintaining energy.

The process of shifting was predefined in the two equal primordial particles of half positive and half negative forces, for even in these bearers of cosmic energy, the whole of creation was contained as movement, dynamism, activity and evolution. Consequently, the shifting into two-thirds positive and one-third negative forces had to take place to attain a dynamic motion, which now determines the rhythm of infinity and allows the forming and creating forces to flow in infinity.

I repeat: The shifting of the forces was necessary as the driving force for creation with its movement, activity and evolution of the universe, because only limited motion is possible between like-vibrating poles.

The Father-Mother-Spirit is the giving and receiving principle in one. The two-thirds positive force, the paternal part, is the giving principle. The one-third negative force, the maternal part, is the receiving principle. The interaction of these forces produces the love-stream. In the primordial powers, the love-stream intensified and began, first within itself, to prepare the structure and form of creation.

The seven basic powers of God are also called as follows: The first four basic powers are the natures of God, the creative forces. The further three basic powers are the three attributes of God. They are the powers of filiation that raise to filiation the nature beings, which developed and took on form in the heavenly mineral, plant and animal realms.

*Infinity is in a state of continual
expansion and evolution*

All of infinity is a potentiating perpetual motion: The Primordial Central Sun, which consists of two-thirds positive and one-third negative primordial power, causes its energies to flow into the All via the seven prism suns. There, the primordial powers are absorbed by the spirit beings and by the spiritual minerals, plants, animals, nature beings and stars and planets.

The primordial power is harmony and constant motion. Everything that it can fully permeate remains in harmony. In this way, everything that is pure is in permanent unison and in motion.

Since every movement produces new energy, more energy than was released flows back into the primordial mass. This causes the interaction between the positive and negative force in the Primordial Central Sun to increase, because from infinity the seven times seven forces again flow together in the Primordial Central Sun and become one stream, the All-power. This then flows, in turn, into the seven prism suns, the suns of the natures and attributes. These split the one stream, the All-power, into the spectral lights of infinity, which, in turn, flow out into the All again. Through this process, all stars, spirit beings, nature kingdoms, souls and human beings are in continuous motion.

According to a predetermined cycle, a part of the energy is again taken back by the Primordial Central Sun where it is potentiated and then flows again as one stream, the All-power, into infinity by way of the prism suns. In this way, the purification planes and the the partly and fully material worlds also receive the primordial power, the Holy Spirit, according to their spiritual development, to their existing spiritual potential.

*The emergence of perfect creation
with the pure forms of Being
after a few pre-creations*

The divine principle, the giving and receiving, is the self-potentiating perpetual motion. Through this, infinity, too, is in a state of continual expansion and evolution.

At the beginning of creation, this took place on a small scale. Through the constant breathing in and out of the primordial energy, the Spirit brought and continues to bring about the continuous expansion of infinity and the evolution of the forms of being. In this way, the perfect creation of the heavenly worlds emerged.

Because of the increased motion of the two equal poles in the Primordial Central Sun, and because of the rearrangement of the primordial energy into two-thirds positive and one-third negative power, the primordial energy multiplied. Again and again, the All-Spirit let a part of this primordial energy flow into the All and began to "model" with this ether light. Several "pre-creations" were necessary before the "model" was fully developed, and the All-Spirit, who then was also the Father-Mother-God, granted full life to His model.

The constantly intensifying pulsation of the primordial power out into the All caused turbulent-like movements. The ether light, the forming spirit mass, flows from the Primordial Central Sun, the primordial light. The All-Spirit took a part of the ether light to model. Another part of the ether light was poured out as creating and forming power. This creating and forming power of ether light is not omnipresent power, but energy for shaping the spiritual form.

With the intensified activity of the two equal primordial particles, an ever-higher potential of energy developed. During the pre-creations, in which the Spirit brought everything into harmony and unison in the ether light, the re-arrangement into two-thirds positive and one-third negative energy occurred. At the same time, the All-Spirit, the intelligence, the primordial energy, deliberately had a part of the negative primordial energy flow into the All to the forming ether light. A part of the highest light intensity of negative primordial power was now in the forming ether light. This portion of omnipresent negative power gave cause to the Fall.

Through the perfect creation, every created and begotten spirit being received a quantum of this omnipresent negative primordial power. The first created and begotten spirit beings received more than those that were begotten after them, because the first spirit beings had and have the greater radiation power.

The first spirit beings accepted the omnipresent negative power, and thus became spirit of His Spirit. However, it behooved them to assimilate this part of the negative omnipresent power and to voluntarily transform it into creating and forming energy, thus bringing themselves into the primordial stream as children of God. By doing this, they voluntarily surrendered their claim to omnipresence and acknowledged the sole omnipresence of the Father-Mother-God, the Creator of infinity, who had beheld, created and brought them to perfection through the spiritual procreation. The spirit beings thereby accepted their filiation and activated in themselves the filiation attributes of Patience, Love and Mercy. At the same time, they acknowledged the primordial energy, the Father-Mother-God, as the sole omnipresent primordial principle.

In this way, the Father-child relationship came into being. The children became the image of the Father in form and shape. However, with their light-potential they were and are not omnipresent, but only All-conscious. This means, they can behold and grasp everything in their consciousness, and can move here and there. This also means that they are free in all of infinity.

As I briefly revealed before, the Father-Mother-Principle came into being through several pre-creations, which were attempts toward complete creation. The ether light, flowing energy, had to gradually find its way into the energy that had taken on form. This took place by way of the pre-creations.

The rearrangement of the half positive and half negative primordial power into two-thirds positive and one-third negative power took place over the course of eons. During these eons, the All-Spirit breathed out again and again, shaped the ether light and breathed it in again, until creation was fully fermented and resembled the primordial harmony, the vision of the All-Spirit.

Through this "weaving and plaiting" of the Father-Mother-God, by rearranging a part of the negative primordial energy—whereby inconceivable movement developed through the ether flowing within and without the primordial light—polarity also developed. This polarity came forth from the Father-Mother-Principle, the giving and receiving principle. The Father, the two-thirds positive power, is the giving principle. The Mother, the one-third negative power, is the receiving principle. This is why the Father-Mother-God is in the one energy, the primordial energy, in the omnipresent power.

The beings created by God and the first procreations should voluntarily bring themselves in as children of the Father-Mother-God, and thus become images of the Father who are free and independent, however, not omnipresent.

The first highest light-intensities, the first-created and begotten children—except for a few—agreed to be beings of the Absoluteness, but not omnipresent. All those beings, who were, as yet, unable to take this step toward the filiation, although accepted into His love-stream by the All-Spirit, the Father-Mother-God, were nevertheless not received as heirs of infinity. He left them their freedom and gave them eons to decide.

However, to all those who accepted and received Him as the one omnipresent Father-Mother-Principle, He consciously granted free will, and installed them as heirs to infinity. And the still undecided beings were given the free will to reach a decision over eons—but not yet the heritage of being conscious children of infinity.

Despite the indecision of some beings, the ever-larger growing creation was populated with light-beings by way of spiritual procreation. Every being had within itself a quantum of omnipresent energy, which it should voluntarily transform and bring itself into the primordial stream as the child. This implied the recognition and acceptance of the Father-Mother-Spirit as a unit and the sole omnipresent power. A large part of the spirit beings, both male and female principles, accepted the filiation and polarity. In the still undecided spirit beings, the quantum of omnipresent negative power was mostly latent.

The Father-Mother-God accepted into the filiation all created and begotten children. But into the seven basic powers, He received only those who had contributed the quantum of negative omnipresent primordial power to the filiation forces of Patience, Love and Mercy. Thereby they became free from will and could call every cosmic energy their own and use it lawfully.

*The manifestation of
the omnipresent primordial power,
the Father Ur or God-Father—
His spirit-dual, the highest female principle*

The All-Spirit had already given Itself form during the pre-creations. The foreshadowed form of the Father and the foreshadowed form of the Mother emerged from a part of the ether light during pre-creation. Therefore, merely an outline form of the Father and an outline form of the Mother existed in the pre-creations: two not yet perfectly modeled spiritual figures.

In pre-creation, the spiritual worlds of the animals and plants were also forms that had not yet been fully fermented. However, since the All-Spirit breathed into the pre-models, the

56

indicated, not yet fully complete, forms again and again, until they were absolute—also the indicated form of the Mother went back again into the omnipresent primordial energy.

However, in the absolute creation, the omnipresent primordial power was and is the Father-Mother-Principle in one.

The manifestation, the eternal heavenly Father, the Father Ur, is the Father of all the children. Therefore, He is the sole being that in its radiation is united with the omnipresent law and simultaneously unites the two poles, Father-Mother, in the omnipresent eternal law. The eternal Father is called the Father Ur because He unites and represents the primordial powers, the Father-Mother-Principle, in one being—in the Father Ur.

Standing next to the Father Ur is not the Ur-Mother as a being, which likewise represents the omnipresent negative, that is, the maternal part. At the side of the Father Ur, who likewise bears within and radiates the omnipresent negative power, the Mother-Spirit, stands His dual.

His dual does not bear within the omnipresent power. In the basic powers of the Spirit—Patience, Love and Mercy—it is the child, because the three filiation attributes characterize the children of God as beings.

*Mentality, polarity and duality,
the equally vibrating forces
of drawing, creating and procreating*

Mentality, polarity and duality exist in creation. Equally vibrating forces attract one another. Polarity as well as mentality and duality are forces that attract equally vibrating energies that then unite and act together according to their kind of vibration, whether polarity, mentality or duality. Duality brings forth the spiritual power-potential for further children of heaven. The duals, the positive and negative principles, again beget together spiritual children for whom they are the paternal and maternal aspects. However, above all is the

58

Father Ur, the manifestation, which embodies the Father-Mother-Principle in the omnipresent energy of the law, in the primordial power.

The manifestation of the Father Ur also took a dual who was and is on an equal footing with all female spirit beings, except for the quantum of negative omnipresent primordial power, of which the Father Ur transferred more to His beheld spirit dual than He transferred to all other spirit children, because she had to be like Him in vibration and radiation, since like power-potentials attract, in turn, like power-potentials. God-Father, the manifestation of the primordial power, that is, the Father Ur, has the highest light-potential in all of infinity, more than all of His children, regardless of whether they are male or female principles.

The spirit dual of the Father Ur had no advantage over all other spirit beings. The dual of the Eternal, of the Father Ur, also had to transform, that is, bring in, the quantum of omnipresent negative primordial power transferred to her and prove herself as a child among the children of God in the three attributes of Patience, Love and Mercy.

A brief summary

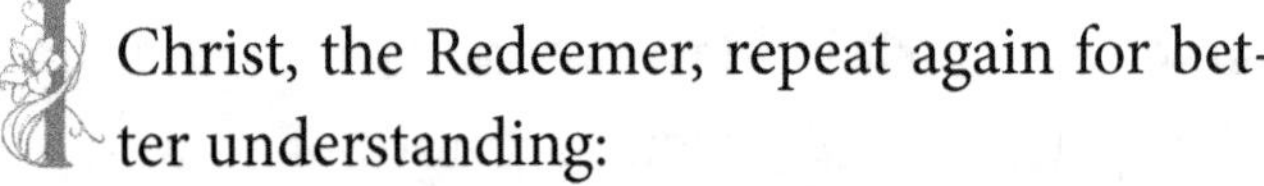

Christ, the Redeemer, repeat again for better understanding:

The Father Ur breathed a greater quantum of omnipresent negative primordial power into the first created female principle than into all other spirit beings, including those that were begotten during the later course of the event of creation. For this reason, the first female angel received more omnipresent negative primordial power so that she was matched with the potentiated power of the Father Ur.

This explains the spiritual principle: Like attracts like. Spirit beings with like or similar aptitudes in the seven basic powers, for example, having similarly vibrating aspects or predispositions in the basic power of the nature of Will—in other words, who have an equal amount of potentiated energy from the basic power of Will, thereby complementing one another more strongly—will then work together in their spiritual tasks for the whole. This is polarity and mentality, the attraction and communication of like forces.

If a duality results from the altogether equally vibrating forces of polarity and mentality, then the male and female principles work together more intensely but nevertheless in unity with all beings.

The first-created female angel may have accepted her share of the filiation, the quantum of omnipresent negative primordial power, but did not absorb it, because she did not bring her share of omnipresent power into the flowing All-Power, into the Father-Mother-Spirit. She could not get over the fact that she could not represent the omnipresent maternal part as omnipresence.

Those who as beings during the course of creation brought their share of negative primordial power into the Father-Mother-stream attained absolute free will for all eternity in all of infinity.

Such a being is aware of everything. By virtue of its All-consciousness, the spirit being can move in all the spheres of infinity. It is not excluded from any lawful possibility, since, by bringing in the omnipresent negative primordial power, it has become the law itself.

The principle of drawing, creating and pro-creating includes free will. Over the course of the eons of eternity, God gave His own the possibility to bring their share of negative primordial power into the omnipresent stream. Although the first female principle had not yet brought her share of negative primordial power into the omnipresent stream, the Father Ur still took the first, and most beautiful in radiation female creation as His dual, to show as a living example what is expressed in creation in all the natures and forms: the mentality, polarity and duality, the equally vibrating forces of drawing, creating and procreating.

For the one who is the law everything is possible. It has freedom of movement in all infinity. The spirit being beholds in itself the heavenly planes with their stars, beings and nature kingdoms. It can either linger in itself on a certain plane or be elsewhere with a speed that cannot be explained in human words.

When God Father transferred to His first-beheld, partly created and begotten Son a portion of the omnipresent positive primordial power and appointed Him Co-Regent of the heavens according to the eternal law, the quantum of omnipresent negative primordial power, which lay partly latent in the first female principle, started to become active. The spirit dual of the Father Ur wanted to be like God, omnipresent in the flowing energy, in the same way as the first Son is omnipresent with Him in the four natures of God.

The first female principle now realized more and more that as child, daughter and dual, she was placed on an equal footing with all sons, daughters and female duals, the sole exception being that she had a higher light intensity than all other female principles.

The negative sensation of wanting to be like God ripened more and more in the highest female being. The highest female being did not want to bring her quantum of omnipresent negative primordial power into the filiation attributes, because in this one part of omnipresent, negative primordial power, she saw the possibility to become omnipresent once again in the divine omnipresent stream. As the female principle, she wanted to be equal to the first-beheld Son, the Co-Regent. And so, the female angel felt disadvantaged, because her former, now manifested, power-potential, which she should transform into the filiation and dualship, and which was once a part of the omnipresent primordial power, was no longer omnipresent.

*The highest female angel rebelled against
the Absolute Law and won other spirit beings
to her cause. She refused to be a dual
in the filiation capacity*

The disappointment of no longer being able to be in the omnipresence and—despite persistent efforts—in not being received in it anymore caused the Fall-thought to slowly ripen in the highest female angel. She rebelled against the Absolute Law. Inspired by the desire to be omnipresent with her part of the inheritance, she tried to win over many spirit beings—both male and female principles, to her plan. The highest female principle stirred up the part of omnipresent negative primordial power in many spirit beings of heaven, especially in those who had only conditionally or not yet entered the filiation. But she also stirred up the Fall-thought in some spirit beings who had already brought their part of the negative primordial power into the omnipresent stream. Those beings who felt addressed and touched by the first female angel shared her attitude and joined with the first female principle.

After a relatively long life in accord with the divine laws within the time of grace of the eons, in which she should bring in the negative primordial power, the first female principle rejected the dual in the principle of filiation, because she wanted to be like God, that is, omnipresent, equally vibrating in the positive and negative force.

With this revelation about the initially equal forces of the half-positive and half-negative primordial power up to the creation of the eternal forms of the Being, I, the Spirit of truth, have given only a brief insight, so that the person can learn to understand better the law of cause and effect, of sowing and reaping, and the seeker of truth can learn and understand why it came to the Fall, and why the first female angel wanted to bring her part of omnipresent negative primordial power back into the All-power, from which she had streamed forth and become the forming, drawing, creating, procreating and receiving power.

*Christ foiled the intentions
of the Fall-beings*

If the first female principle had been successful in her intention to be like God—omnipresent—then all spiritual forms would have dissolved, because that part of the negative power which constituted the filiation would have flowed back into the primordial power. The dissolution of all spiritual forms would have re-established the original principle of equality: half positive and half negative power.

Even to this day, the idea of equality (half positive and half negative power) still exists in Eastern teachings, because all the details about God's final act of creation are not known. This is why many people, particularly those of the East, cannot accept the Co-Regent, Me, Christ, and thus, also not accept the part-power of the primordial power, My divine heritage, which is the redemption of all souls. This is why, particularly in the East, the view of the dissolution of all forms still exists, even today.

The Fall, also called the fall of angels, ensued from this event of creation, and is a still existing turbulence. Its vibrations were condensed to such an extent that it became solid substance, called matter.

Through the part-power of the primordial power, the power of Christ, who I Am, all souls will attain purity again and through this, find their way back to the divine unity, whereby God leaves them the free will.

Through My divided heritage, which is effective as a spark in every soul, the dissolution of all forms was prevented. I, Christ, the Redeemer of all souls, will restore the absolute cosmic unity through My heritage, the part-power of the primordial power—according to the eternal plan of creation.

The part-power of the primordial power, the power of Christ, is active in the law of cause and effect and will remain in force until all souls have left the wheel of reincarnation. The four spheres of purification form the wheel of reincarnation.

The soul's path of evolution out of the law of sowing and reaping begins with the actualization of the eternal laws.

In the incarnated souls, in human beings, My Redeemer-power works more intensely than in the disembodied souls that are in the spheres of purification. At the same time, the grace that pours into soul and person offers protection to the willing soul and to the person striving for perfection. The protection given through My increased grace is necessary for those striving toward God, particularly at the beginning, when the God-willing person takes the first steps on the path of evolution toward God. On Earth, people with different degrees of consciousness live together in a very small space, which, however, also means that the danger of burdening oneself is very great. People living in such confined spaces strive for purity and chastity—as well as people who indulge in immorality, who send out aggressions and insult their neighbors when they do not do what they want.

Matter is the manifestation of negative thought forms and, as seen from the Spirit, it is illusion, that is, transitory

Over the course of the millions upon millions of years, the turbulence caused by the Fall-beings became ever denser. The unlawful feelings and thoughts, the wanting to possess, to be and to have, took and still take shape in the form of condensed radiation, that is, matter. The strongest form of crystallization—matter— is nothing but the manifestation of thought forms. They were brought forth through the wrong world of feelings and thoughts of the Fall-beings—but also of the spirit beings who wanted to rush to help their brothers and sisters, the Fall-beings, and then became entangled in matter.

Matter, the coarse-material, as seen from the Spirit, is merely relative and not reality. It is illusion, not reality.

The part-material worlds and the purification planes also emerged through the Fall-thought: to want to be like God without being divine.

God is omnipresent, and divine is the spirit being, which, through its high consciousness, beholds and experiences within itself everything that befalls and takes place in infinity.

Christ gives this revelation
to awaken souls
and human beings to life

So that ever more souls and human beings recognize themselves and learn about the origin of their life and experience it in themselves, I, Christ, the Son of the living eternal Father, the Co-Regent of the heavens, the Redeemer of all souls and human beings, reveal Myself. So that souls and people learn to correctly understand and accept the laws of love and of life, I give increasingly deeper insights into the eternally prevailing law, the life.

And this revelation from My Spirit should again give insight into the life of the Spirit and help many souls and human beings gain inner freedom and a life in the Spirit of My Father and theirs. Souls and human beings should become aware of the power of feelings, thoughts, words and deeds, which shape their lives, and which can make them free—or can bring them hardship, misery, worry and illness, depending on how the soul feels and the human being thinks and acts.

Human beings are the builders and architects of their own fate. Their feelings, thoughts, words and actions are the building blocks for a happy life—or for a life of hardship, misery, illness and suffering. Whatever is present in the soul, light or shadow, will be made manifest to them in one of their lives on Earth.

My revelations should be recognized and understood according to their meaning, so that deep wisdoms may come forth that express far more than the letter itself. The word as such ex-presses little. The vibration that flows into the word from Me, the eternal Spirit, allows the deep wisdoms, the truth, to be recognized.

What the human being is able to grasp and understand from My words, which are vibra-tions, awakens the soul and the human being to a life in Me, the Spirit. The human being be-comes receptive for the eternal truth, because the one who is of the truth knows My voice.

My sheep know My voice.

The multiplicity that the Almighty beheld in its entirety, and that He brought forth from the unity, remains, lives and works in unity, in the great whole.

A part of this multiplicity—which lives through the law of unity, recognizes itself in the whole and knows it is secure there—is all the forms of life: the eternal pure creation with its heavenly nature kingdoms and the pure heavenly beings, the spirit beings, as well as part-matter and full-matter and the planes of purification with their beings, souls and human beings. All this is part of the unity of God.

The manifested thought form, the material garment, the human being, brought about the trinity, spirit—soul—body. This trinity exists only where part-souls or burdened spirit beings, that is, souls, have incarnated—that is to say, animals that have a part-soul and human beings who bear within a fully matured soul as the bearer of life.

What is not incarnated, what does not live in a material garment, does not consist of this trinity. Stones and plants have no soul. They are vivified by divine rays of life. Stones and plants are called "duos." They consist of the spirit ray, or spirit-rays, and the shell, the external form.

All pure spiritual bodies of the beings of heaven are duos. They are a bi-unity: spirit, which means flowing divine energy, and energy that has taken on form.

The development of the pure spiritual body occurs through the compression of ether and the potentiation of the spiritual form. From this, a spiritual particle structure gradually emerged, and continues to emerge.

In the worlds of heaven, the compression and potentiation begin with the spiritual mineral kingdom and continue through the kingdoms of plants and animals until the balanced form of a nature being attains the filiation of God: the pure spiritual form, the pure spiritual body, also called ether body. The primordial power, the life, the primordial energy, also called divine energy, is in this ether body.

Without the primordial energy, God, both spirit body and human being would not be viable. In the same way, all material life forms, such as stones, plants, animals and human beings, cannot exist without the primordial energy.

In the pure spiritual kingdom, the bi-unity exists, the duo: spirit and spirit body. The human being consists of a tri-unity, also called trinity: the spirit—the primordial power—the soul and the physical body.

The entire universe, the visible and the invisible universes, exists because the primordial energy, God, respirates and maintains it. The law, the love, consists of the four natures and the three attributes of God. These seven divine basic powers are the all-maintaining principle, also called the primordial energy, God, or the Holy Spirit.

All pure spirit forms are the essence from the primordial energy and have within all the forces of infinity. Everything is spirit of His Spirit. The eternally maintaining principle, the Holy Spirit, is active through the created forms, through the ether body and through all Being.

The Fall-thought transformed down a part of the primordial energy that had become form, parts of spiritual planets, and with them, the collectives of stones, plants and animals. Over the course of time, during which further negativity followed, the transformation of the highest energy into lower vibration, into matter, brought about the law of cause and effect, the law of sowing and reaping, also called the causal law.

As the envelopment of the spirit body, the human being, gradually formed, the trinity came into being: the Spirit of God in the ether body, now called soul, and the envelopment, the human being—hence, spirit, soul and human being.

The envelopment of spirit and soul, the human being, is subject to time and therefore, transitory. Everything that is not of a pure, fine-material structure does not last in the long run.

All Being is based on energy, on radiation and vibration. The pure heavens with the pure spirit beings and the spiritual mineral, plant and animal kingdoms, matter with its forms and human beings, the part-material spheres with their part-material beings and life forms, the planes of purification with their souls—everything is vibration.

The pure spirit beings have insight into all spheres, those of the pure heavens, as well as of the soul realms and of full matter. All other beings, such as the souls in the planes of purification, have insight only as far as it corresponds to the development of their consciousness.

People who are totally focused on matter see only matter and its kind. People who seek and open the Kingdom of God in themselves and have risen spiritually above the four planes of purification, that is, vibrationally, recognize and behold the true laws in themselves. They have insight into what takes place behind matter and the planes of purification. They have awakened to the sonship and daughtership in the spirit of infinity.

Thus, once a person's soul has reached this expansion of consciousness and traversed the four planes of purification, that is, once its consciousness is in the filiation of God, it will then be apparent to soul and person what lies behind matter: the mode of acting and living of the Spirit.

The pure forms are self-luminous. They are not irradiated by a sun as is the human being.

The primordial power radiates into their inner being and through them.

On the other hand, the material universe and thus, the physical body, are irradiated from without, by suns and planets, and therefore, not permeated. Only then, does matter become visible. If light did not irradiate bodies and objects, there would be no reflection and all things material would not be visible. A disembodied soul can perceive and live only in those spheres that it has activated as light and energy in itself.

In the soul as well as in the human being only so much becomes perceptible as they have activated in light and power. A soul can reflect what it has actualized on its journey to the light of God. In the soul only that radiation can become effective, which it has again opened through the actualization of the eternal laws. This is then expansion of consciousness.

If a soul is still very tied to the Earth, then it is also denied the view into higher and lighter spheres, since it has not yet developed the higher frequency of vibration of these spheres of life.

Its consciousness is therefore still restricted. The higher spheres do not find any reflection in it yet, since they are still covered by its burdens.

If there are karmic bonds with higher spheres, the still lower-vibrating soul is occasionally granted a glimpse into lighter spheres through a temporary supply of energy. The still existing karmic bonds—perhaps with a higher sphere—are seen within by the soul. In this way, the soul is stimulated to forgive or to ask for forgiveness.

This insight into higher spheres takes place as follows: Through increased radiation, provided by the planets which guide it and under whose influence it still is, the soul's consciousness is temporarily expanded. Within its own consciousness, the soul sees the still existing burdens. With this, it is led to recognition—to forgive or to ask for forgiveness.

A similar process takes place in an incarnated soul, in the human body. Soul and person mature only through self-recognition, actualization and forgiveness. Both the soul in the spheres of purification as well as the human being are urged again and again by the eternal law via the causal law, the law of cause and effect, to recognize themselves and to strive for a life according to the law of love. The more limited souls and human beings are, the more the people are tied to their own world of conceptions. In many cases, people then fail to hear the call of the eternal law because they are living according to their own opinions and thus, often against the eternal law.

The pure beings, on the other hand, live the law and are therefore themselves the law itself—self-luminous. Nothing can cloud their spiritual primordial sensation. They behold all things in the right light, thereby recognizing all processes in their entirety.

The pure, the absolute, does not affirm the limitation of time and space. That is why limitation cannot exist in the long run. God may well see the limitation but does not affirm it.

For the pure being, the pure consciousness, everything is open and clear. The pure permeates everything, including matter, all suns, worlds and human beings. We see matter as solid substance. However, as everything in infinity, it is vibration, energy.

Spiritually blind and deaf people
do not know their true being and
can no longer perceive God in themselves

The pure sees and affirms the Being, but not the appearance. As long as people are still bound to people and things by desires and ideas, they also remain bound to time and space, and their true being remains hidden until they make an effort through self-examination of their true origin and of their true being—to see things as they are and not as they seem.

If they succeed in examining and experiencing themselves, they will no longer interfere in the laws of nature. They will see human beings as the image of the eternal Father and respect life—the life of their neighbor and of their second neighbor, of the plants and animals, of all of nature. Only then will suffering, hardship, disease, hunger and spiritual death come to an end.

What people sow, they will reap. Those who violate the ironclad, universal law act against themselves. Many people go on sowing ever more causes. For each cause that has not been repented and settled in time, the effect will follow.

Many people have built and continue building onto already existing causes of hatred, envy, suffering, destruction, illness and all other adversities and plagues. In the individual, this produced, and still produces, a narrowing of consciousness, through which soul and person no longer could and can perceive the primordial sensation, the Spirit of God, the voice of the Almighty.

Therefore, God, the eternal law, can guide only a few people directly. All other people are guided by God, the eternal law, through the causal law—what a person sows, that person will reap.

A great number of people and souls have become deaf and blind to the word of God. In this spiritual deafness and blindness, people seek contact only with their own kind, and, in so doing, forget that they are beings from God, and therefore, divine. The soul, however, consciously or unconsciously seeks the origin of the source, until it has immersed in it again.

People have their language. They speak the language of the country in which they live. The words of people are sounds, that, strung together, produce language. They are merely an aid, but never the communication of the pure forces of the soul with God.

Because of their externalized way of life, of which language is a part, many people have become spiritually blind and deaf. This is why the language and the voice of God is unknown to them.

Since many people can no longer perceive the holy primordial sensation, the word of God within, in their soul, I, the Spirit of life, reveal Myself through the mouth of a human being, through an instrument called by Me, in the word and in the mother tongue of the instrument.

The word of human beings is limited. Therefore, it is not possible for Me to reveal in their entirety the all-encompassing laws of life and the law of cause and effect, in which the whole event of the Fall is reflected.

I, your Lord, the Spirit of life, Christ, lead you back to the holy primordial sensation, to God, to the word of God, to the truth. Thus, may all those who hear and read My word, given through My instrument, endeavor to understand the spiritual meaning, so that what is revealed by Me may become a true enrichment for soul and person.

In this world of external forms, everything is relative. Whatever human beings observe with their physical eyes is limited. As viewed from the perspective of the eternal consciousness, it is merely illusion, and thus, unreal.

The earthly world is an expression of the senses and thoughts of the individual. This means that the world consists of thought forms. It will be transformed, as will all that is coarse-material, because the eternal law produced and produces only what is ethereal, that is, self-luminous.

Everything that is not the Absolute Law is viable only to a limited extent, and therefore, non-existent in the Spirit of God.

God is Spirit, the highest-vibrating energy of love and life. God beholds everything in its perfection, purely ethereal. Since God is absolute, highest vibrating energy, only the spiritual, the pure ethereal structure, which is absolutely translucent and without shadow, can exist in the long run.

The thoughts and projections of all generations of humankind, from its inception until now, are reflections of things past and present. Whatever a human being has once caused and still causes that has not been redeemed, that is, that has not been transformed, characterizes the respective epoch.

Just as people, each individual, are the mirror of their soul, in the same way are the events of history of each era, each epoch, the mirror of those who lived in an earthly garment in former times and now live again in this present epoch. Through the qualities of the soul they brought with them, they shape the world view and what happens in the world.

*The indirect guidance of God works
via the law of cause and effect
and via the heavenly bodies.
The spiritual consciousness diminishes
in those who go through their days
oriented to the world*

People who live merely a world-oriented life and are not conscious of God are guided indirectly by God, the eternal law, via the heavenly bodies.

The primordial power, the source of love and life, is the energetic power in all celestial bodies for spirit beings, souls and human beings as well as for the nature kingdoms.

Only as much energy flows to the changed, transformed-down atomic structures of the part-material suns and planets, including the Earth's sun as well as all material suns and the purification spheres, as it corresponds to the respective evolution and as can be received by souls and humans through the actualization of the eternal laws.

Due to the inconstancy of individual persons and the vacillations of their consciousness—one time Spirit, then again world, one time spiritual striving, then again falling back into the world where, in turn, even more burdens are awaiting them—the irradiation of the primordial power constantly changes. This means that according to the state of development of soul and person, the primordial power flows more or less abundantly, also depending on how the scale tips for each individual, toward the spiritual or toward matter.

Thus, if people fall back into a sensory life bound to matter, the primordial power in them decreases: their spiritual consciousness constricts, and thought forms—thought constructs they created themselves—begin to influence them. These, their own thought forms, can then be transformers for souls that are similar in vibration to their thought forms—or also for other people's thought forms or for forces from the atmospheric chronicle that vibrate in the same or similar way. All these can then influence soul and human being.

Those who are not on their guard and carelessly let day after day go by, who do not monitor their thoughts and do not counter the negative thoughts, the thoughts of hatred and envy, jealousy and self-love, with positive, selfless, constructive, that is, lawful, thoughts, waste their precious life energy. They live, and do not know why. Their earthly garment dies, and their soul does not know where the journey goes. They leave this Earth and are strangers to themselves—and will also be somnambulistic strangers even there, where their soul is heading.

The ones who are a stranger to themselves because they live far from God, considering only the world as their habitat, who do not ask about the cosmic laws or apply them to themselves, will keep asking the question: Why are there natural disasters, hardship, illness, worries, problems and much more?

God is the Absolute Law.
The pure heavens and the pure
spirit beings are also the absolute
all-encompassing law of life.
The seven basic powers of life

Those who read or hear My word must start from the assumption that God is Spirit and that all pure forms of life have come and still come forth from the Spirit. Therefore, God is all-knowing Spirit, primordial energy.

The word of God is the primordial sensation that finds its expression in all Being and in all beings—also in those human beings who have drawn closer to the primordial source, the Holy Spirit, in their inner being.

The primordial sensation, the flowing, communicative consciousness, is also called the All-sensation. It is the expressive power of the law. The law, God, is eternally flowing energy.

In its manifold facets, colors and forms, the primordial sensation, the eternal law, is the rhythm of infinity. It is action and reaction and, at the same time, is expressed in the spirit beings and in the entire creation.

The primordial power flows from the Primordial Central Sun, from the two primordial particles, the positive and the negative power.

The primordial power consists of the seven basic powers. For this world they are called Order, Will, Wisdom, Earnestness, Patience, Love and Mercy.

These seven basic powers, which are the life of all Being, flow into seven prism suns, which orbit the central heavenly body, the Primordial Central Sun. These seven prism suns, also called secondary primordial suns, split the seven basic powers into seven times seven energetic powers.

These seven times seven powers, the law of God for all Being—for spirit beings, souls and human beings, for the mineral and nature kingdoms—are the all-encompassing law of life.

The seven basic powers, split into seven times seven rays of life by the prism suns, are the lawful principles for a life in infinity. Each ray of life is a law-ray, which is effective as a lawful principle in infinity.

God is Absolute Law. Since everything is the law, God, the pure heavens, too, are the law, God, as are all spirit beings who inhabit the heavens.

The eternal law also maintains the causal law, the law of cause and effect.

*The direct guidance of God can be attained
only by those who have found their way
out of the causal law, of the wheel
of reincarnation, and who have again
become the Absolute Law*

The causal law is energy that has been transformed down, which resulted from the causes of all Fall-beings, of all burdened souls and people.

The Absolute Law streams through the causal law and guides all souls and people who are still bound to the law of cause and effect, according to their causes. This is the indirect guidance.

94

People who have found their way out of the law of cause and effect and thus out of the wheel of reincarnation, through the actualization of the eternal law, attain the direct guidance of God because they are immersed in the Absolute Law, God.

Through the Fall, a part of the pure primordial energy was changed and transformed down. This transforming down of the primordial energy went so far that a degree of crystallization developed in the universe, which is called matter. The Earth, this part of full matter, is the dwelling place for the incarnated souls, the human beings.

Every soul in the spheres of purification, as well as every soul in the earthly garment, is called upon to develop spiritually and again become what God gave to the pure beings: the Absolute Law, which it became and is.

However, as long as a soul keeps incarnating in an earthly garment, it brings along its still existing all-too-human stirrings and inclinations and, in its thoughts and actions, continues to work on situations and tasks that it had not completed in one of its former lives. This may happen in a different epoch with quite different means and possibilities. But still, the soul continues to work on them and on its own thought complexes until they perhaps take on material form and shape.

Only once soul and person awaken to spirituality, will they begin to put their life in order and to gradually overcome the many self-created thought forms and burdens of the soul through Me, the power of Christ. In this way, the soul becomes pure again—and through Me, its Redeemer, it can be led back to the Absoluteness.

God gives love unceasingly, even through the causal law, also for the Earth, for every soul and for every human being. From the basic law, the immutable law, from God, the seven times seven law principles, which are like spectral colors, flow unceasingly. They vivify soul, person and all Being, which is in the law of cause and effect.

*Human consciousness is limited to time
and space and considers the earthly existence
to be reality. Only a spiritually awakened
person recognizes the transitory
nature of matter*

Repeatedly, these seven times seven divine powers, the law principles of God—which will transform all that is condensed and raise it to purity—were once thwarted by the Fall-beings and now by human beings, through their negative thoughts, words and deeds.

In this epoch, few people and souls have developed themselves out of the causal law. Most people violate the Absolute Law on a daily basis and continue to create causes under the causal law.

Since many former Fall-beings did not fulfill the Absolute Law, and over the course of time, many people have violated and still violate the Absolute Law, intersections developed over billions and billions of years, both in the planets and in their atmosphere. Different radiations, vibrations, colors and forms then emanate from these points of crystallization. The result of this—from one epoch to the next—is the different insights, perspectives, orientations and impressions.

Despite these differences in epochs, the soul returning as a human being always begins at the point where it stopped its development during one of its former lives—until it awakens in My Spirit and consciously allows itself to be guided by the law of love.

I repeat: Everything is based on vibration. Even matter with its structure and the inhabitants of the Earth, the human beings, are vibration.

The vibration of the physical body is mostly in accord with the Earth's frequency of vibration because both, human being and Earth, are matter, potentiated, crystallized energy.

Matter has its measures and weights. In human terms it is a real solid substance, cosmically conditioned and integrated into the great totality, having its function in the universes, in infinity. This viewpoint is relative, because the three dimensions of matter, oriented to space and time, are a part of the causal law, which is indeed embedded in infinity, but is kept within certain limits by the eternal law.

For those who limit their consciousness, their thinking, feeling and wanting only to the dimensions of time and space, reality is the material life, the earthly existence. But those who, through spiritual striving, through the fulfillment of the holy laws, approach the inner kingdom—of which I said "the Kingdom of God is in you"—will see matter in its relative existence: They know that it is subject not only to change but also to transformation.

The spiritually awakened person knows that the physical body is of this Earth and has been created only for this Earth—that it is merely an instrument or a vehicle for the spirit body, the soul, that dwells within. But much becomes possible for the spirit body, the incarnated soul in the human being, once soul and person strive toward higher ideals and values in the course of their spiritual development, and also put them into practice.

Values that are not related only to this world, but are in the right relationship to matter, that are more spiritually oriented than merely materially colored through the glasses of egocentricity, bring about equanimity and peace. A mature soul and a person who is in alignment with the inner kingdom, with the Kingdom of God, will learn more and more about the laws that eternally prevail and to which matter is also ultimately subordinate.

*The disembodied soul experiences
matter, space and time as unreal*

At night when the body is asleep, the mature soul gathers deep knowledge and impressions from higher spheres. It takes these with it into its earthly garment, however, overlaid by the receptivity of the mind, which is meant only for the three-dimensional world.

On its "journey" into timeless spheres, the soul learns that matter is unreal since time and space do not exist in the eternal law. It experiences that without a body it can penetrate space and is not bound to time.

Something similar happens after the disembodiment of the soul, after its physical death. According to its spiritual development and maturity, the soul proceeds to those places where it finds the same, that is, what corresponds to it, what is similar to its nature. The disembodied soul, the fine-material structure, is able to pass through all the spheres of vibration that it has opened in itself. This means that whatever it has attained through a lawful life is evident in it—and it can also go there.

The alert soul will recognize that the possessions that were once its own while in the earthly garment are no longer solid matter. It passes through everything it once called its own while in the earthly garment, through all that it cherished and cared for, and that were solid matter for it. Suddenly it finds that worldly things are no longer concrete—no longer solid matter. What was once reality for it as a human being is now no longer concrete. It has become unreal because the soul is now in another aggregate state.

If even an alert soul can gain this insight and pass through time and space, through all solid matter, how much easier it will be for a pure spirit being to penetrate everything—since its home is infinity, pure, fine-material substance.

*Those who act against the cosmic laws
or modify them create dissonances
and changes in all spheres of life,
in and on the Earth*

Every negative thought and every unlawful action always had and have a limiting effect on those who have thus turned away from the eternal law. The sum of all transgressions against the laws resulted in limitation and condensation and, over the further course, in crystallization, in matter, space and time.

It would be possible for human beings to change the material structure and to gradually lead the condensation back into higher spheres of vibration, because the highest powers are inherent in them. Human beings are called upon to vivify these forces and to apply them lawfully.

In this way, the material structure would be refined, because the seven basic forces of the universal law would become effective and would gradually lead the entire material structure into another aggregate state. However, this could be accomplished only through those people who change their thinking habits and their way of living, and who actualize the eternal law of love, of peace and unity.

The four elements, fire, water, earth and air, make up the respiratory system of the Earth. If people continue to interfere in this lawful process, the whole organism of the Earth will be disturbed over the course of time. This would have an influence not only on the Earth's magnetic fields, but also on the magnetic currents, which are the law of the Earth and the planets, and which belong to their solar system.

Seen as a whole, every disturbance also has an effect on the Earth's axis.

Every change in and on the Earth causes, in turn, a change in and on the human being, in and on the animal world; it triggers a corresponding reaction in the plant world and even changes the radiation of the minerals and stones.

What happened in prehistoric times is happening again at the present time: Those who modify the seven basic powers of infinity through wrong thinking and unlawful action not only create dissonances in and on the Earth, which, in turn, result in ever new changes, but also in themselves.

Over the course of time, the continuous interactions, the dissonances in all life forms—which changed forms, colors and sounds—influenced human beings, the nature kingdoms and the entire solar system. Through unlawful behavior—whereby the cosmic forces were misused—polar shifts, eruptions and the like developed again and again. Right up to the present time, the Earth has not and does not come to rest.

Therefore, whoever interferes with the cosmic laws and modifies them inevitably creates dissonances in all spheres of life on Earth and in the Earth itself. Since every thought, every word and every action is energy, and since no energy is lost, everything positive, such as lawful thinking and acting, as well as everything unlawful, falls back on the originator, on the human being and their soul.

Just as every person has a spiritual substance within, which is called soul, so does every life form have its bearer of life, the Spirit. The Earth, too, the dwelling planet of humankind, has a spiritual substance. It is called the Earth-soul.

The Earth-soul, a spiritual part-planet of heaven, was and is unaffected by the changes in the Earth's crust. Therefore, it is merely the network, the material shell, the Earth, which changes, and not the soul of the Earth.

The Earth-soul, the spiritual part-planet, does not accept the negativities of human beings. A person's soul, however, absorbs the positive as well as the negative. This means that a person's soul can burden itself, but not the spiritual part-planet, the soul of the Earth.

The "book of life," therefore, is the soul of a human being. The soul registers both the positive and the negative thoughts, words and deeds.

Only the originators of what is negative on Earth can burden themselves, but not the innocent life forms: the minerals, plants and animals that God gave His children for the preservation of their material shell.

Human beings, minerals, plants and animals should form a balanced relationship: Harmonious radiations should emanate from all life forms, radiations that would complement and strengthen one another and contribute to the well-being of humankind. However, this is not the case, since human beings have created dissonances in themselves and in the nature kingdoms. Therefore, every unatoned cause will be followed by its echo, the effects—in and on the Earth, as well as in and on the human beings. What has been and is inflicted on the Earth by human beings will fall back on them.

*There is a continual interaction
between the energy field and
the magnetic field
of the human being and the Earth,
in which the law
of cause and effect takes place*

Human beings are bundles of energy that, according to their thinking and acting, create their own energy fields or magnetic fields. Therefore, every person has their own energy field and magnetic field, which correspond to their way of thinking and acting.

There is a continual interaction between their magnetic fields and the magnetic fields of the Earth: The reactions of the Earth are transmitted to the people through the interaction between person and Earth, just as the actions of people are transmitted to the vibration of the Earth. Whatever human beings do to their Earth, to their dwelling planet, they do to themselves because of this interaction between human beings and the Earth.

The law of cause and effect works and is effective in every human thought. The seed already lies in every stirring and inclination. As long as people are still under this causal law, their thoughts, words and deeds are, in turn, the result of their correspondences, their causes.

Therefore, whatever people do to their neighbors or to their second neighbors, the animals, and to the Earth with its nature kingdoms is what they will reap themselves. The magnetic fields of the Earth register all the actions of the inhabitants of the Earth, the human beings. And the magnetic currents—which are the sound-carriers of the great "Earth-man," the Earth—bring all resonances, no matter what their fallout, whether positive or negative, back to the one who emitted them: the human being.

Whatever people do to their neighbors or second neighbors is engraved in their own soul. It is absorbed by their book of life, by their soul. Since everything is based on vibration, they accept and absorb the vibration they once emitted, and are still emitting.

The Earth's magnetic fields register every dissonance, especially the human acts of violence that provoke considerable atmospheric disturbances as well as disruptions in and on the Earth, for instance, by nuclear tests and the like. All dissonances are transmitted by the magnetic currents, the sound-carriers of the Earth's magnetic fields, which may also be figuratively called the nerves of the Earth.

The magnetic fields of the Earth are ranges of varying frequencies which, in their entirety, are called the Earth's magnetic field. They are the "nerve points" of the Earth, and, at the same time, the mirrors of the dwelling planet. If these mirrors of the Earth are altered and dulled by humankind's wrongdoing, then this has an effect on the entire Earth: on the climate, on the nature kingdoms and on the people. The magnetic currents even change the behavioral pattern of the animals.

Human beings are influenced according to their thoughts and actions, because they are, to a greater or lesser extent—depending on their state of consciousness—connected to the total magnetism of the Earth. Just as in many cases, animals change their instinct and often become unpredictable, it happens in a similar way with people bound to the Earth. The elasticity of the body decreases. They become depressive and aggressive.

The plant world also changes its characteristics. Many highly developed plants are dying out and lower species are emerging.

*The negative, destructive forces emanating
from human beings weaken the forces
of their own soul and body, and lead to
blows of fate and illness*

Harmoniously balanced magnetic currents would be beneficial for a person's weak nerves. They could restore and strengthen a weak organism. Decisive, however, is the person's attitude toward the Earth.

If people are in harmony and thus in accord with life, then they will also reap harmony. Harmony is the same as "symphony," which means it is the accord of soul and body. Harmony is an uplifting and stabilizing force for soul and person. Whoever leads a life that is positively oriented in thoughts and words, whoever strives to attain unity with all forms of life will also absorb the positive forces, activate them and strengthen them in themselves.

The opposite happens when people develop negative, destructive forces. The negative, destructive forces will influence them, stimulating them to further unlawful acts. Over the course of their life or lives, this causes soul and body forces to weaken, so that indispositions, blows of fate and illnesses take the place of happiness, contentment and health.

However, if the behavior of people is positive, both toward their neighbor and their environment, they will attract the still existing positive energies from the magnetic currents. These will, if necessary, then restore and strengthen their own magnetic field.

In the earthly existence everything is relative. Whatever is negative also has positive aspects in it. Those who lead a selfless, positive life are also able to recognize the positive in the negative, to affirm and enhance it. And whoever activates the positive forces will, in turn, be served by the high, noble and pure energies.

Therefore, recognize that the spiritual law of attraction for spirit beings, souls and human beings is: "like always attracts like" or "like draws to like."

Those who live under the law of cause and effect should reflect every morning on the fact that every cause and every negativity, be it in feelings, thoughts, words or deeds, creates causes. Every cause already bears in itself the seed of its effect. A new cause can, in turn, develop from an effect, if people do not recognize the effect in time, thus continuing to violate the immutable law. But if they recognize in time the effect of the cause that they have themselves set, if they repent of it and try to make amends for the negativity, the effect need no longer follow—or only to a minor extent, depending on the nature and intensity of the violation.

What people sow they will reap. And, whatever they do to the great "Earth-man," the Earth, will also fall back on them.

The Almighty said: Subdue the Earth. He did not say: Exploit it and maltreat life, the plants and animals. Even the stones feel the harmony and disharmony of human beings! Therefore, it is the obligation of human beings to promote the positive energies, to apply them sparingly and in the right way, according to the eternal law of love and unity.

For example, changing the atom, its fission and application, is against the law of love and of peace. It is against the All-harmony, God.

Whatever triggers disharmony is negative and therefore already bears in its cause, in its predisposition, the seed of destruction. Every dissonance, no matter when, where and by whom or what it was triggered, disturbs the harmony and contributes—generally speaking and in relation to the majority of human beings—to disturbances in all areas of life.

Just as harmony or disharmony is registered by the Earth's field and is transmitted to the sound-carriers, to the nerves of the Earth, to the magnetic field, in like way, it is propagated in the animals and, in particular, in the highest creature on this Earth, the human being. The nerves of human beings become tense, the life energies wane and they fall ill. Because of the low intensity of light of soul and body, the organs become receptive and susceptible to illnesses, viruses and harmful bacteria.

Thus, unlawful vibrations gave and give cause for increased tension in both the nervous system and in the organs. The blood circulation, in particular, is considerably disturbed in the process, which, in turn, gave and gives rise to certain illnesses.

Blood is the carrier of material life. If the blood is not in order, then the entire organism may be affected detrimentally. If the Earth, with its forests, oceans, lakes and rivers, no longer produces sufficient oxygen that is needed by human beings to breathe, then the consequence is the contamination of the blood—and as a result, the organs are weakened, and they have little resistance. Since the blood flows through the whole person, impure blood simultaneously affects several organs and other substances of the human body.

Every illness has its cause.
It may have been created in a former life
on Earth. The soul brings with it
the positive or the negative aspects
that it acquired in its previous lives

Every indisposition and illness has its cause. The cause must not necessarily have been created during this life on Earth. Whatever comes into effect in this incarnation flows out of the soul. Therefore, the cause of an illness can flow out of a burdened soul, which, in the

116

repeated transition from birth to death, has laden itself with ever new burdens.

A soul can incarnate and go through many earthly lives in the human garment until, through self-recognition and actualization, and by accepting My deed of Redemption, it walks the spiritual path of purging and cleansing its base ego, thus increasing the Redeemer-light effective in it. Sooner or later, every soul and every human being has to undergo the purging of the soul—either in this life on Earth or in further lives or as a soul in the spheres of purification, in order to again become the conscious image of the eternal Father.

Those who do not master their life, who do not ennoble their nature add new causes to the old, over and over again, even if in different ways, depending on the life habits of the time period in which the soul again incarnates, bringing with it the unatoned sins from former lives.

Thus, the newly incarnated soul radiates what it has acquired in former lives. Its aura reflects its good and bad thoughts and deeds. They are the memories and correspondences. They determine the inner attitude toward life, from which people think and act. In doing so, people build up new thought forms and, according to their behavior, attract the same again.

People who in former lives thought and lived in a worldly way and focused only on matter will go on thinking and working in a similar way in their present earthly existence until they awaken to spirituality and gradually change their way of thinking.

What the soul has affirmed and promoted in a previous life on Earth and what is still unatoned is further promoted and built up by it in this existence. Scientists, for example, then again try to split atoms to gain nuclear energy. Physicians strive again to continue working with organ transplantations, and churchmen again pursue different-minded people. Thus, the same and similar things are continued again and again by the same souls—only in other human bodies and with another external form, but characterized by the same radiation. In this way, the souls in further existences on Earth build again and again anew on the structure of their fate. One cause follows another, and one effect after another becomes active.

People who cleave to the world will counter Me, the Christ, with the following: We have to carry out experiments to be able to maintain life on this Earth, because people need food, clothing, coal, electricity, oil and many raw materials and other resources, to make life as comfortable as possible. We need—thus speak people who cleave to the world—motors, airplanes, ships, vehicles and much more, so that we can move forward faster. We need medications and hospitals. We need houses to live in. We need factories that produce food, clothing and many other things. We need all this and more to be able to live.

My answer, the answer of Christ, is:

Raise yourselves, O humankind, to spirituality, so that your spiritual horizon may broaden, and you may apply and administer the fullness of God, your spiritual heritage, in the right way.

The heavenly bodies and the nature kingdoms show how human beings can live. Nature has given and gives itself in manifold ways. But human beings raise themselves above the gift, which is nature, and want to be independent of it. The heavenly bodies show people how radiation can be made useful and how energy can be produced.

On the one hand, human beings strive for independence; on the other hand, they tie themselves to their achievements, which—as they can now realize—will not serve them in the long run, because everything that cannot be brought into harmony with the laws of nature will be the doom of humankind.

If people are self-centered, that is, centered solely on themselves, this means that they are also oriented to this side of life. This is why they do not recognize the countless sources that could bring people a healthy and happy life, nor do they experience them.

On the other hand, God, who is the abundance, serves those who make the nature kingdoms and the firmament a part of their living, thinking and acting, who respect and cherish life in all its manifestations, whether plants, animals or minerals. They will recognize and experience what a great treasure dwells in and around them.

This treasure from the Spirit, the fullness, can be recognized and received by people only when they have proven themselves as cosmic beings through the actualization of the eternal laws. Then the forces of infinity will serve them. If they accept these thankfully, by living a life in the Spirit, possibilities upon possibilities will reveal themselves to them, which they could use for their benefit and well-being.

For this, the person first has to change: from being a person who is oriented toward the world and cleaves to the world, to someone who thinks in a spiritual way and is oriented toward the divine—a person who acknowledges the source of all Being and also lives according to the eternal cosmic laws.

Humankind has turned ever more away from God, its Lord, turning to external things and values and its own achievements. In so doing, the intellect was overrated and the trust in God, the highest power, was largely lost.

Many people live like pagans. They have their idols, their gods, which they revere. The first one is the "god" Mammon, who has made people its servants and slaves. The other gods are prestige, power and the drive for recognition.

Only a complete reorientation,
a turning away from material living and
thinking and turning back to spiritual
values could change the world

The time is near in which it becomes more and more evident that neither church leaders nor statesmen and scientists can save humanity. For this reason, ever more people will again turn to the belief in a higher power and find support there.

The great of this world and their adherents will be unable to halt the impending world chaos, despite ever new measures and precautions, which only lead to further entanglements. Whatever they do and deem good and beneficial leads to further entanglements—and thus, to further causes, which already anticipate the effect in the seed.

Alert people will recognize this and mend their ways. Those who sleep will fall into their self-dug pit.

All those who cleave to the world are biased and view events only from their own perspective and in a way that might be useful to them as human beings. Biased people are prisoners of their own ideas and desires.

Everything temporal is subject to change, and worldly people are subject to their ideas. Those who acknowledge only three dimensions are limited in their thinking. They can, in turn, pass on only what is limited and do only what is human. People who think only in stereotypes will take up the idea of their predecessor and expand on it according to their own stereotypes and thought patterns. With their thought pattern they can possibly influence many people and even initiate a new epoch—which, however, still bears within the seed of causes from a previous epoch. Thereby the radiation of the Earth can change as well as the convictions of the people who live in this epoch.

Only the fewest inhabitants of the Earth can imagine that a life according to the laws of infinity is able to express itself in completely different aspects than those of food, housing, clothing, electricity and the exploitation of natural resources.

The fullness of the great whole is, as essence, in all things, in every human being, on and in the Earth and in the firmament. However, humankind must first be awakened and raised to spiritual recognition. It must first recognize and strive for the inner ideals and values to be able to come into its spiritual heritage. Only then can the undreamt-of possibilities open up that lead to health, happiness, peace and love. As in heaven, so it could be on Earth.

For this to happen, there must be a complete change of thinking on the part of those responsible in this world, but also on the part of the majority of the people.

It is written, "The Kingdom of God is within, in you." The Kingdom of God can come to this Earth and become visible only when every single human being opens the Kingdom of God in themselves.

The egocentric three-dimensional view of the world changes in those people who live according to the eternal laws; it becomes universal. People who are able to think and live universally draw from the source of inexhaustible life. They become creative and work for the benefit of many.

People who do not try to reach the basic principle of life, God, and do not strive for spiritual customs and morals remain biased toward the world, controlled by their drives and passions. With their crude character, their coarse nature, they shape the world and with those of like kind lead it into material ruin.

If all people were to strive for the refinement of their five senses, their character, too, could become more refined. The world would be more perfect, and the people healthier. Then there could be peace among the people. Then life would be completely different. Everything that characterizes the worldly people of today, their wanting to have and to possess, could be transformed into a life of community and unity. In this way, the world would be spiritualized, and the power of God could visibly take over the leadership.

Human beings are children of God endowed with free will. Through the filiation of God, it is possible for them to influence both on higher and lower ranges of vibration, all according to their way of thinking and acting. Thus, by virtue of their way of thinking and acting, they can have an effect on different ranges of vibration, each of which corresponds to their mental and physical sphere of influence. They can influence both the positive and negative forces. The positive forces that they develop and assimilate build them up and result in health and well-being. Negative forces influence them and others. They reduce their mental and physical vigor, and this, in turn, has its effect on corresponding vibrations in others.

As long as the inhabitants of the Earth remain pleasure-seeking individuals, striving only for the satisfaction of their passions, for money, prestige, possessions and culinary pleasures, there will be no peace on this Earth, and the world will not look any better. On the contrary, people will fight one another more and more. Their continuing wrongful behavior will make the Earth barren. Humankind—that is, each individual—would have to become more frugal so that a change of mind could take place among the nations.

If people find their way to a spiritual evolution, to a renewal and change of their hitherto egocentric life, they will dissociate themselves more and more from present human achievements, from the world of high technology, from culinary delights and from passions. However, the more removed people become from the divine stream, the less spiritual vitality they have. As a result, they automatically turn to external things and seek diversions in the world, since their inner life has become impoverished. They no longer have access to the realm of the inner being and, therefore, need ever more external sources in order to live. They also need more food and encroach on the world of animals, becoming butchers and carnivores. They indulge in alcohol and nicotine and increasingly slide down into a passionate life.

However, if the law, the life, becomes ever more strongly effective in a human being, the spiritual fullness in the soul, the heritage of God, also awakens. It is the strength for a true, higher and modest life.

Those who strive for higher ideals and values, for the fulfillment of the eternal laws, will not only intuitively learn and experience what humankind and the nations truly need. Above all, they will be led and nourished by the primordial source, which is My Father.

Through the lawful way of thinking and living of many people, their environment would also change. As soon as the surroundings of the individual change toward the positive, the dwelling planet Earth automatically also comes into a higher vibration. The result of this would be more highly developed life forms in the plant and animal kingdoms. The plant world would change. Higher forms with greater light intensity would radiate on soul and person, awakening further positive forces of healing and life in human beings. The animal world, too, would change and increase in its power of light. The Earth would yield more vibrant and larger and healthy fruits, with considerably more nourishing substances for soul and body.

The forces of the Earth could give the undreamt-of to humankind—a life of happiness and peace! Healthy and harmonious people would be with one another and subdue the Earth in the right way.

Thoughts are powers. Positive, divine thoughts and lawful actions change not only the Earth's radiation toward the positive and constructive, but also that of the entire solar system. Through humankind's positive orientation toward the divine, the entire solar system could be raised in its vibration. What has a higher vibration also receives increased powers from the eternal law, God. The spiritual development of humankind would bring about a change from the lower to the higher. If individual people had put in order the seven times seven spiritual powers effective in them—the fullness from God—by living a pure life, and were thus able to draw from them, unimagined possibilities would be given to them. The actualization of the eternal laws would have resulted in the direct guidance by the Spirit of God and, consciously to them, God would be among His own.

However, as long as the majority of people orient themselves solely to the world of earthly appearances, to people with earthly abilities and qualities, the Earth's radiation will be changed more and more and the vibrations will be transformed down—both spiritual and physical, as well as the vibrations of the planet Earth. In this way, the entire radiation of the Earth changes more and more.

*What was inflicted on the Earth from the
start falls back on the perpetrators.
The group karma of humankind*

Whatever the inhabitants of the Earth have done to their planet ever since it came into existence and has not been atoned for has an effect on the perpetrators. Either their souls expiate it in the spheres of purification or they continue to return into an earthly garment with their causes, until these have, for the most part, been settled.

If the thinking and senses of the inhabitants of the Earth stay cleaved to the world, then they will build up new burdens on their already existing ones again and again. They create thereby causes over causes, not only in themselves, but also on and in the Earth.

The causes may be manifold. They can be negative thoughts of hatred and envy, or defamations and disparagements. These causes are then expiated by the souls as effects with people whom they have to serve, or with people with whom they have to spend their whole life, because they once failed them or sinned against them.

Negative actions can be committed on and in the Earth. For example, through nuclear processing and nuclear testing. Such causes have wide-ranging effects. They have an effect in and on the Earth, in oceans, lakes, rivers and underground watercourses, in the atmosphere, in human beings and animals.

By merely approving these grave causes, a person shares the guilt for everything that had to suffer from them. This is then a "collective karma" or "group karma," a karma shared by a large number of people.

Everyone should ask themselves: How does our dwelling planet Earth react to all those people who do not respect it, but instead pollute it, thus maltreating life? All people should ask themselves whether they are also a part or want to be a part of this collective karma!

Many scientists, for example, search and research only in the material realm. They see in the material being the only reality and the only possibility to be able to collect experiences, in order to eventually become famous. The further, and for them invisible, spheres of life, the sustaining force, which is the life in matter, which sustains the material and carries the forms—that is, the law that is effective behind matter—is considered by only few. To many, the invisible force, the Absolute Law, is a thought-image of the mystics, which seemingly cannot be realized.

As long as human beings do not examine what they actually are, they will know themselves only by their external appearance. This means, they do not know themselves. Those who do not know themselves merely want to be confirmed in the world, thereby creating cause after cause.

The human being, however, is a cosmic being that bears within a spiritual body called soul. The soul cannot be measured or weighed, since it is purely spiritual and does not relate to the vibration of material energy.

The eternal law—that is, the life, which is effective behind matter, behind the three-dimensional world—becomes accessible only to those who first examine themselves and recognize who and what they are. Those who strive to actualize the eternal laws that are effective in human beings and in all Being and apply them correctly in the world and on the Earth will draw from the divine Wisdom and find their way to the inner truth.

They will then become true investigators, genuine mystics, who, through the fulfillment of the divine laws, penetrate the depths of their consciousness, from where they receive intuition and revelation, in order to achieve for humankind and the Earth what would be necessary for the Earth and humankind to be healthy and for peace to pervade the world instead of hatred, envy, conflict and war.

God is energy. God is spiritual atomic power; human beings can investigate it, and it can become effective through them.

Once the energy, God, becomes effective in human beings, it radiates through them and works through them for the benefit of many.

When people violate the earthly laws, they are sentenced to punishment, either to a fine or imprisonment in jail. Those not with God are against God. They "scatter—and gather coal" for themselves and for many who believe in them and do like or similar things.

Something similar holds true for soul and person when they violate the eternal law: The consciousness of the soul diminishes. It is superimposed by the human ego. The people are egocentric. They are thus a prisoner of their own ego. Their ego-bias forms the prison bars through which they look and see only what they consider right, good, and true. Their ego sees the world just as it sees itself and how it expresses itself in the world. In this way, worldly people fashion their world, thus influencing their environment.

The more intellectual the individuals are, the narrower their consciousness. They are prisoners of their ego.

The leaders of the nations, as well as the scientists and theologians, must change. As long as they join hands and support themselves in a worldly way, the nations themselves and the individual people on the Earth will achieve little, because the external power determines them.

There are few great ones of this world who endeavor to examine the spiritual laws and discern the instructions of life by which humankind might attain health and deliverance from its imposed yoke, and thus escape its fate. People who cleave to the world will only cause difficulties for themselves and their fellow people. Whether they are scientists or theologians, such people are not true scholars and therefore, not the true mystics who can explore and see the depths of life! As long as the dancing around the golden calf, around possessions, prestige, honor and money does not cease, there can be no better world to sustain and nourish the people.

However, a new humanity will awaken! Many people will change their way of thinking. They are the shapers of the spiritual human race that lives in friendship with the Earth and sees it as a great living organism, which is willing to serve humankind by nourishing it.

The Earth, a living organism,
is built by cosmic radiation.
All unlawful actions change the radiation,
create disharmonious frequencies
and disturb the balance of the forces
in all life forms on the Earth.
Nuclear reprocessing, soil displacement,
exploitation of natural resources,
shifting of the Earth's axis

The living organism, the Earth, is built by cosmic radiation. This, however, requires all the substances in the Earth that form the breeding ground for the radiation, which then penetrates and maintains and fosters life.

This is the eternal spiritual principle: In all of infinity nothing can be transformed or formed if the eternal power, the immutable law, is not effective. If the substances of certain metals and minerals and the like were not present in the soil, the cosmic radiation could not fertilize the planet Earth; it could not support growth, and thus, it could not stimulate the substances in the Earth to propagate. This is why it is a serious violation when human beings exploit the Earth and undertake massive displacements on it. Through this, they change the cosmic radiation in and on the Earth.

Everything should grow organically, but people interfere with life again and again. They crossbreed species of plants and animals at will. They are inventive and endeavor to bring forth ever new species of plants and animals. Over the course of time, this results in a completely changed radiation, because the Earth, too, like all other planets, is a radiation form that is oriented to the cosmic life, to the radiation of God. Human beings, too, are a cosmic form of radiation. If they change this radiation through unlawful thoughts, words, and deeds, they fall ill. As long as people do not change, as long as they do not think and live cosmically, they will experiment over and over again, because their souls are searching for what they lost in many incarnations: the light, the purity and beauty.

Every unlawful form of action changes the cosmic radiation within the sphere of the Earth. For example, the many corners and edges of buildings as well as of furniture break the cosmic radiation. Every angular object changes the vibration and the vibrational frequency in itself and, depending on the material, creates disharmonious frequencies in a broad area. Seen as a whole, these altered energies have, in turn, an effect on human beings and on the nature kingdoms. Even the so-called skyscrapers, which are meant to serve the people—the world population is expanding and the buildable land is getting expensive—set free the vibrations and forces that influence not only the city in which they stand, but also the atmosphere, which, in turn, affects the people.

Recognize, O human beings, when the scales are in balance and you suddenly put or even throw a brick on one of the scales, what happens? The scales will tip heavily to one side, and if you throw the brick on the scale pan, the device may end up being bent or even break.

Recognize, O human beings, this is similar to what you are doing to your Earth. The task of the Earth's axis is, among other things, to keep the Earth in balance. But what do people do? With negative and aggressive forces, they influence the scales of the Earth.

People have some knowledge about radiation. Despite their knowledge about the dangers threatening the Earth through many different causes such as nuclear reprocessing, rock quarries and excavation, they continue to exploit the Earth without second thoughts.

The long tunnels through the mountains and the hollowed-out coalmines also cause a change in the Earth's axis. The result of such mass shifting of soil and rock is a change in the Earth's radiation as well as the Earth's axis.

Human beings exploit the Earth's oil reserves and process them with other substances out of which they produce various products that they—as they believe—need to live.

143

What can a perforated and partly hollowed-out planet be good for? What do the scales of the Earth look like?

In their sum total, the many large and small causes have an enormous effect on individual persons. Those who do not strive to preserve or restore harmony, the accord of the forces in themselves, will suffer from this.

The sum of all negativities is the cause of illness, suffering, hardship, misery, hunger, epidemics, catastrophes and wars: What human beings have sown and are sowing, they will reap.

Human beings endeavor to explore everything that is still unknown to them. They want to understand the external things, thereby forgetting the central point, the life, the Spirit, that sustains all things and is the moving force in everything.

Unknowingly and thoughtlessly people carry out earth displacements and the like, by which they also change the atomic structure of the Earth. Thereby, material atoms come into a changed light intensity. Through this, the vibration changes of the material atoms—which are ultimately the building blocks of the Earth.

The material atoms hold the Earth's structure together and establish the relationship to the cosmic irradiation. If this is disturbed, because the vibrational frequency of the atoms has changed due to displacements of earth or a change in the atomic structure, then there are inevitable dissonances in the Earth's interior and on its surface. The effects of these disharmonious forces make themselves felt accordingly in the nature kingdoms and in human beings.

However, the very foundation of all Being is the Spirit. A material atom, is nothing but a crystallized spiritual atom which, over the course of billions of years, surrounded itself with differently vibrating forces by displacements or changes of the radiation intensity.

The material building blocks, no matter what they are called, whether atoms, molecules or elementary particles, are nothing other than divine energies that have been transformed down. The light was crystallized through wrongful feeling, thinking and acting. It is called matter or solid substance.

What is not salutary for a person is not beneficial for the Earth either. And what is not good for the life of the Earth is not beneficial for the human being either. After all, the human being is a product of this Earth and thus, identical to it. If the Earth is sick, then the product, the human being, also becomes sick.

In the following example, you will be able to recognize how people treat the Earth, the vast organism, which is the source of sustenance for human beings:

A surgeon performs an organ transplant in a person, which, according to the eternal law, is just as unlawful as experimenting in and on the Earth. After the organ transplant, the patient has to take the most varying kinds of medications so that the body does not reject the foreign organ.

The foreign organ in the patient is a foreign vibration. Sooner or later, the physical body will react—even if it is years later, when the organism of this person has become immune to the medications. Complications set in; the body tries to reject the foreign organ.

With this example, O human being, you can see that when two different kinds of vibrations are brought together, this will always lead to dissonances.

Therefore, whatever is added to, or taken from, the Earth's organism on a daily basis, has its effect on the natural body, the Earth, and on the perpetrator as well, the human being, who is a product of the Earth.

The Earth, the great "Earth-man," is abused daily by human beings. In a figurative sense, the Earth, too, has its organs and circulation: the oceans, lakes and rivers, the water veins, the magnetic fields, the North and South Poles, the nature kingdoms and much more.

Figuratively speaking, this means that people are constantly carrying out "organ transplants" in and on the Earth. The consequences of this are being experienced by people daily anew, in and on the various continents.

Each continent has its own particular magnetic field, which, depending on the metals, ores and all the mineral resources found there, emits vibrations that are transmitted by the magnetic currents to the entire Earth and everything that lives on it: human beings, animals, plants and stones.

If considerable amounts of mineral resources are exchanged from continent to continent and subsequently modified, that is, refined, processed and applied accordingly for various purposes, then the intensity of radiation of the continents from which they were removed, as well as on which they were stored or processed, changes.

You, O human being, have heard that the magnetic currents are the sound-carriers of the Earth's magnetic field. Because of these sounds—which are vibrations like everything else—the structure of the Earth likewise changes. Every sound affects the characteristics and genes of human beings and animals to a greater or lesser degree, depending on its intensity and tone. Plants and minerals also react to sounds. All changes, which started from the Fall-thought of the Fall-beings and continued to take place in the further course of the latter's condensation into human beings, were and are registered by the entire Earth and, therefore, by the circulatory system of the dwelling planet, its water veins.

Humankind as well as all the animals of the air, of the Earth and of the waters are dependent on the vibrations of the planet Earth. All Being reacts to sounds, colors and forms. Just as human beings behave toward the Earth, so does the echo return to them from the Earth.

The extinction of many animal and plant
genera; the change of instincts

Through the unlawful influence of human beings on the nature body, the Earth, many animal genera have become and are becoming extinct, and other animal forms with other characteristics, in turn, are developing anew. It is similar in the plant kingdom. Many plants are becoming extinct and other species appear whose effects are not yet known to human beings. The disposition and characteristics of people have different effects in each epoch.

Humankind is living in a constantly changing Earth and Earth-atmosphere. The dissonances triggered by people, whether in colors, forms or sounds, also have a disturbing effect on the nervous system of those whose vibration is on the same level of radiation.

Through Me, people are called to spiritually transform themselves upward through noble convictions, so that they may be enriched with true insight and a true life. Since the soul of a person is not of this world, it is possible for the soul, as well as for the human being, to set out on the path of evolution in order to draw from the cosmic life and to subdue the Earth in the right way.

Every dissonance, whether it is emitted by the Earth or comes from the burdens of human beings, has an effect in manifold ways. An irritable, disharmonious person tries to relax in various ways. For example, by eating or drinking more, or through increased sensuality. In their diversity, these signs and their effects indicate a broad spectrum of negativity and increase the base inclinations in the person.

Worldly people take each day as it comes, without consideration for their neighbor or their second neighbors, the animals and plants. Higher ideals and values are foreign to people who are oriented to the world and think only of themselves.

As a result of the interference in the laws of nature, the instinct of the animals, which I,

Christ, call the life of sensations, is changing. It changes from epoch to epoch, since human beings constantly change and subordinate themselves to the mindset of others.

Domestic animals, in particular, suffer under the treatment of people and their opinions. They in particular change their way of life, because people influence them as well as their genes. Many animals are intimidated and irritable. Their instinct is totally oriented toward matter and the world of thoughts of human beings. According to their mentality, and after thousands of years of faulty development—and as a result of the crossbreeding of animal species—animals have adopted many human habits.

Among the pure forms in the spiritual nature kingdoms, there was no drive to fight and devour one another, just as there is no aggression and hostility among the pure spirit beings. It is a result of the condensation of the Fall-beings— that is, of their distance from their purpose, which brought about their degeneration—that animals are hostile to each other and fight and kill each other just as human beings do.

This means that over the course of their development, and according to their characteristics and imprinting, many animal species took on the same inclinations as human beings. The vibrational field of many animal species resembles that of many human beings.

Even the deceitfulness of human beings can be found in animals. For instance, the cuckoo lays its eggs in another bird's nest, and the magpie eats the eggs of other birds. These two examples are not the only ones. The unkindness of human beings, which knows no bounds, now prevails in a similar way throughout the animal kingdom.

Each form of life has, according to its spiritual development, its own energy potential, a magnetic field. The human being as well as the animal, the plant and the stone radiate the degree of consciousness that corresponds to their energy potential. The human being calls the dawning of consciousness the radiation of the degree of consciousness or aura.

Only human beings change their aura. According to their way of feeling, thinking and acting the aura changes in color and shape.

As a result of the wrongdoing of human beings toward their neighbor and second neighbor—the animals, the plants, and, seen as a whole, also the planet Earth—the Earth's magnetic field and the magnetic currents are constantly disturbed. This results in various tensions in the magnetic field of human beings as well. Likewise, animals, plants and all other forms of life suffer from the dissonances in the Earth's magnetic field. And over the course of time, these dissonances cause further negative tensions in human beings and animals.

If the magnetic field of the Earth is disturbed and the dissonances in the magnetic fields of human beings and animals are increased, this then has an effect on the genes of human beings and of the animal world. This leads to a wide range of illnesses.

The role of the nervous system in the development of illnesses and blows of fate

The solar plexus, a central nerve complex in human beings, is an important switching point in the nervous system. It can be considerably influenced. If this switching point, including the nervous system, is detrimentally affected by dissonances of various kinds, illness and blows of fate may be the result.

Dissonances develop with sounds, for example with glaring or dark colors, with thoughts of hatred and envy, with quarrels, with brooding and aimless thoughts, with severe problems and worries, with thinking about things long past, with the inability to forgive or with other difficulties that a person cannot let go of.

Those who allow themselves to be driven by their thoughts and desires and are preoccupied with their problems day after day lose the orientation to what is noble and beautiful. They see themselves as misunderstood and suffering. In this apathetic, irritated state, they absorb many contrarious vibrations, negative thoughts, which in many cases are the cause for a burden to become effective in their inner being, which then expresses itself in or on the person as an illness or blow of fate.

Such effects are not physically caused, but psychologically, because the nervous system, the network that links body and soul, became tense, thereby decreasing the life force. This results in an increased emotional movement and may trigger burdens, that is, spiritual causes, which then show themselves as effects in the body.

The nervous system, also called the network of nerves, is of fundamental significance in the development of indispositions, illnesses and blows of fate.

The magnetic currents
and their relation to human beings.
Beneficial and harmful effects
of the rays of the sun

As already revealed, the magnetic currents are the sound carriers of the Earth's magnetic field. If the magnetic field of the Earth is disharmonious, then the magnetic currents, too, are disturbed. This interaction—one time harmony, then again disharmony—also causes in human beings that one time the magnetic currents of the Earth are beneficial, another time they are harmful for them. It depends completely on how soul and person vibrate, on the state of their energy field.

Since everything on the Earth is relative, it is entirely up to the thinking and living of individual people whether the magnetic forces will influence them and in what way. The resonances of the magnetic currents are different in every season, on every day, and even in every hour. This is why their influence on human beings and on the nature kingdoms varies according to their vibration.

Only those people who are themselves disharmonious are subject to the dissonances of the magnetic currents, because only like affects like. Spiritually oriented, harmonious people, on the other hand, will absorb ever less dissonances. As they spiritually mature, it is even possible for them to influence the negative vibrations in a positive way or to neutralize them.

Although the magnetic currents of the Earth can transmit very negative resonances due to constant changes that result from the multiple influences of human beings, certain frequencies are still beneficial to people who have a correct, positive attitude toward life.

People who have a positive relationship with the nature kingdoms can charge their own magnetic field with the positive forces of the Earth's magnetic currents. The positive forces of these magnetic currents are especially beneficial during the early morning hours when the sun brightens the Earth with its first rays. In these early hours of the day, they are more strongly enriched with the Odic force, the healing and life-giving force, because when it is night on the Earth the negative vibrations—the many negative thoughts, words, and actions of people—are reduced while they are sleeping. When the atmosphere has become still, the spiritual power, the Odic force, flows more intensely to matter.

Around midday, the magnetic currents direct more solar particles to the Earth. These penetrate not only the dwelling planet but also human beings because they are a part of the Earth. The conscious absorption of these energy carriers is advisable only when the human being is not directly exposed to strong solar radiation. The midday heat is not good for people's nerves. Too many solar particles may cause considerable unrest. Strong solar exposure causes the nervous system to tense up and gives rise to unrest in the body. It has a detrimental effect on the thyroid gland of the human body, which, in turn, leads to various disturbances in the human organism.

Many solar particles can be absorbed at lakes, rivers and oceans. If it is hot, however, one should seek out the shade. In hot weather there are many solar particles, even in the shade. If they are absorbed correctly—that is, if a person remains in the shade—they strengthen people's magnetic field and stabilize their blood circulation.

The constant changes in the Earth's magnetic field also bring forth animal species that people calls pests or parasites. These life forms, which annoy and aggravate people, are nothing more than the spawn of human thinking and acting and, therefore, a consequence of wrongful human behavior. They are permeated and animated by the magnetic fields. Garbage dumps, polluted waters, radioactive pools, sewage treatment plants, the emissions of nuclear reactors, nuclear waste dumps, sewage and the like are the milieu in which these pests develop.

The human body is a body of thought. Just as people feel, think, speak and act, that is what they are, and that is how they influence their surroundings. According to their way of thinking and acting, they also help shape their time. All people shape and form their environment and the human race of their era. The thoughts and actions of people leave their mark on the time, the world and the fate of nations.

Human beings themselves create the afore-mentioned pests, the parasites, through their wrongful behavior and their negative thinking and acting. Similarly, harmful bacteria and viruses are also products of the wrongful behavior of humankind that may have existed over a period of several eras.

The relationship between an incarnated soul and its respective era. Influences of communities of souls

All human thinking and acting has the following effect: Depending on its burden, the soul keeps returning in an earthly body, in a human body, until it has paid off its debt for the most part. A soul can bring back a large part of its earlier wrongful behavior—the all-too-human emotions, inclinations and desires—into this world, into another incarnation. In the era in which it is again in a new human garment, then, according to its burden, what characterizes this era will have an effect. At the same time, forces—such as the atmospheric chronicle or the same and similar thought forms of like-minded people—have an additional influence on the burdens of the reincarnated soul. They promote the stirrings and inclinations, desires and passions that often define many people in this period.

It is possible that the now incarnated soul, in which certain desires, longings, stirrings and inclinations come into effect and radiate, is one of those people who are striving for like or similar things. If the soul, which has now been touched by these invisible forces, belongs to this group or multitude of like-minded people, then it is part of a group karma that connects these people with one another and that they should resolve together in the world.

This is why, over and over again, two opposing poles are active in this world. Some, for instance, want to use the atom as a source of energy and nuclear weapons because they may have dealt with these in former earthly lives, and may have already done preliminary work for this era. Others do not want nuclear energy. They were opposed to it already in previous lives. They want natural energy, which the Earth gives in rich abundance to those who recognize it and make good use of it.

Or: Some want to support the organization of the Church, because in former lives they were perhaps pope, cardinal, bishop, priest, layman or adherent of this particular religion. Others want to help the Free Spirit to a breakthrough and wish to follow the Nazarene without church dogmas and rituals. They take His teachings alone as the standard for their lives.

Yet another example: Some support this government, others support another one, all according to the body of thought the souls brought with them.

All this and much more is playing itself out on the material plane, in the school of Earth of the soul.

*The soul's cleansing process in the
spheres of purification is more painful*

The spheres in which the disembodied souls live are shaped by similar conceptions, desires, passions, inclinations and interests—all according to what the souls have brought with them from the Earth.

There, the unawakened souls continue to relate solely to matter and live and act in a dream-like state. They cannot create new causes there, because their living and acting takes place only in their dream world and, therefore, nothing is accomplished.

In the soul realm, illness, hardship and worry take shape as images, which cause pain and pangs of conscience to the soul. In the soul realm, the soul experiences in all details what it once caused. The causes that were experienced in images and conditions of pain in the soul realm appear as illness, hardship and blows of fate in the material world.

On the Earth, it is a time of increased grace: It is possible for a soul in the human garment to transfer suffering partly or entirely to its body. Therefore, a soul cleansing can take place considerably more quickly on Earth in a material body than in the soul realms, because during an incarnation there are two bodies that bear the burden: soul and physical body. Moreover, in space and time, grace alleviates, neutralizes and eliminates many things.

In the soul realms, there is neither time nor a second body. There, the purging of the soul is far more painful and takes place in longer cycles. This means that the soul again relives its wrongful behavior in all details, until it learns to recognize itself in this and through remorse, by asking for forgiveness and by forgiving, it accomplishes what has to be carried out so that the images, all those events that it directly experiences, may vanish.

In the earthly garment it is often only memories of unpleasant events, which people mostly do not even remember in detail, or it is an illness that they have to endure, but for which they can be helped, even if only by pain-relieving means.

On the other hand, in the soul realm, there is only the one means for relieving pain: Surrender your wrongful behavior to the Lord, the healing light.

Human beings contract those viruses,
which, in their vibration, are in accord
with the burden of their soul and
the vibration of their body

Thus, the soul brings its baggage back into this world, either partly or completely. In the course of being human, it is touched by the same or like negative thoughts. Through this, it vibrates into people's body, and they become ever more aware of it.

Usually, people will have an occupation that corresponds to their inherent inclinations. The burdens of the soul fall as thoughts into the brain, which has been programmed by a certain activity. People then talk about "intuition" or notions. What then happens is as follows:

First came the thought, then the word. People go to people of like mind and present their idea. If their neighbor takes up their idea, it may be carried out. Since everything created by human beings in the world can exist and be sustained for only a limited time, it disintegrates—for this, there are garbage dumps and sewage plants.

For instance, nuclear weapons and nuclear reactors developed because of such notions.

The contaminated cooling water from nuclear reactors flows into the rivers and lakes and then into the oceans. The final result is an unparalleled contamination of the Earth: Animals and plants die, or animals change their genes and the plants their characteristics. Water turns into a swamp and garbage dumps become breeding grounds for so-called parasites, viruses and harmful bacteria. Like and similar things take place in the lakes and oceans.

In other words: Parasites, viruses and harmful bacteria are the work of humankind.

What people sow they will reap: Parasites are gaining the upper hand. The insecticides used against them as well as the artificial fertilizers may well kill many a kind of life, but at the same time, chemicals promote other pests and new viruses and harmful bacteria. So-called science can hardly register and study them anymore because they are no longer discernible with even the most sensitive technical instruments. They are, in turn, negative forces that affect the genes and—by way of their vibration, the burdened soul—since, as already revealed, everything is vibration. They promote illnesses that are largely still unknown to the people of the present time. Among these are certain types of cancer. Some types of cancer are transmitted by viruses.

The predispositions for such types of cancer were already present as a burden in the person or in the soul. The milieu into which people then enter with their continued wrong thinking and acting causes them to contract those viruses which, in their vibration, are in accord with some of the burdens in their soul. The same applies to the vibration of the body. If it is in accord with certain viruses or harmful bacteria, the body will absorb them. It becomes infected because its genes have a similar vibration.

Therefore, it must be revealed that certain types of cancer are contagious.

Unknowing people fight
all plagues and dangers.
Knowing people recognize and fight
the negative—the greatest enemy—
in themselves

This is why a person has to be reminded over and over again: Pay attention to your thoughts! Strive day after day to monitor and control your thoughts! Surrender the negative, and act in accordance with the law, by sowing love instead of hatred, by sowing good will instead of jealousy and passion! Always have the well-being of people and of the Earth in mind! Then you will do good.

In this way, many things can be neutralized and transformed in your soul. Negativity, that is, burdensome things such as illness and destructive actions, is transformed. You remain or become healthy. Instead of acting destructively, you become a benevolent, kind person who respects and appreciates life.

Just as people can sow negative seeds, which they then have to bear as effects, they can sow in a positive sense, too. Then the effect is an intact and healthy world, where peaceful people live who promote and work for the well-being of all—that is, for peace in this world.

Unknowing people fight everything that seems to them to be a plague or danger. In reality, however, they themselves are the creators of all plagues and dangers. Thus, they should fight themselves, which means to recognize their own desires, longings, inclinations and stirrings and surrender them to Me, the Christ. I Am the positive power that transforms the negative, brightening the world and bringing peace through people who are positive and attuned to the divine. But since people always see themselves as the "best," they declare war on their neighbor.

Only when people recognize that they themselves are the authors of all their positive and negative sensations, feelings, thoughts, stirrings and inclinations, will they take a look at themselves and fight in themselves what they thought they saw in their neighbor.

The neighbor, about whom people get annoyed, is merely their mirror. In their intoxication with the world, many do not recognize themselves—and therefore do not see in themselves the greatest enemy, who destroys the life of the Earth and of their neighbor and ultimately, their own life. As long as individuals do not fight themselves by refining their character, they will always go against in others what they ultimately are themselves.

Thus, people themselves are the pest; they are the virus and the harmful bacterium, because they are the creators of everything that has a destructive effect on the world.

People's radiation shows
what constitutes their soul—
and shows who they are

Unknowing people groom only their outer shell, their earthly body, yet rarely pay attention to their thoughts.

The many human dissonances constantly influence people's nervous system, the network that connects them to their soul. Due to a tense nervous system, My healing and life forces flow into the human body only to a limited extent. This causes mental burdens to break open and body organs to be weakened.

At every moment, the nervous system registers feelings, thoughts, words and actions. Every external disharmony that can vibrate into the inner being of a person, because like or similar resonances are also there, creates disturbances in the body. The result is yet more tension in the nervous system. The consequences are tiredness, listlessness, apathy, quarrelling and dissension. People are no longer masters of their forces. Subsequent consequences are blows of fate and illness.

Therefore, whatever is present in the inner being, in the soul—light and shadow—can be awakened or intensified from without by noise, negative thoughts, by certain thought forms, by viruses and harmful bacteria, by quarrelling and dissension. The effect can then be seen in the body, according to the intensity of what was or is in the soul.

Every cell of the body has a spirit consciousness as well as a subconscious and a consciousness. Via the spirit consciousness of the cell, forces flow into the entire cell structure and reach the organs and the entire body. The cell membrane passes on positive as well as negative energies. Among other things, it affects a person's degree of vibration. Thus, how people vibrate is what they are. Their feelings, thoughts, stirrings and inclinations, their passions and everything that moves them day after day—also their illnesses, indispositions, worries and hardships—are all part of the frequency of their soul.

If, for instance, a person always makes the same mistake, these negative vibrations are registered by the spirit consciousness of their body cells. Consequently, the particles of their soul become shadowed. This is how a soul burden is formed, in the soul and in the soul particles.

In the soul particles, the spiritual atoms form the sounding board. Proceeding from the nervous system, then in the further course, the sounding board of the soul begins to vibrate. The soul comes into vibration and absorbs the vibrations of feelings, sensations and thoughts. It infects itself with the all-too-humanness.

The same takes place with positive forces. If people are harmonious, balanced, selfless and no longer focused on themselves, then these positive forces flow into the soul. There they bring about harmony and peace. In this inner balance, in this harmony and peace, many a soul burden, which would otherwise have afflicted the body through further wrongful thinking, can be transformed or partly eliminated by the Spirit of life.

Every vibration, whether positive or negative, which a person reinforces by repeating the same thoughts, words or actions, finds its corresponding way into the soul, that is, into the book of life. Thus, depending on the person's way of life, the spiritual types of atoms in the soul, in the soul particles, change. With a positive way of life, the powers of the nature of each spiritual atom align with the primordial core of the soul, the core of being, which is the heart of the spirit being.

If a person lives in a negative way, creating one cause after another, the spiritual atoms gradually turn away from the life-giving primordial source, the core of being of the soul, the heart of the spirit being, and turn toward the worldly vibrations. Due to this reversal of polarity from the spiritual to the worldly, to the all-too-humanness, the soul particles become shadowed; for they always expose themselves according to human feeling, thinking and acting. These are spiritual processes that a person can neither measure nor weigh.

What a soul emits and radiates, all that is stored in the soul, form the garments of the soul. These soul garments shape the structure of the human being. It may be delicate or coarse, depending on what lies in the soul particles—impurity or purity, shadows or light, bondage or freedom, the human or the divine.

People's appearance reflects their soul: either beauty and purity or dullness, unpleasantness, even ugliness. A pretty person is far from being a beautiful person. Many people can be pretty. But whether they become beautiful and remain beautiful is already determined by them in their early years.

The human being's outer form and appearance, for instance, the beautiful and noble, the graceful and balanced, are the pure attributes of the soul. The short-lived blossoming of youth, the pretty, is not what the soul brings forth. That is physical. But the radiation of human beings shows how their soul is constituted and, in the end, who they are.

*A person's wrongful behavior changes
the functions of the magnetic fields
and magnetic currents of the Earth*

One thing affects the other and reflects, in turn, what human beings have thought into it or even carried out.

For example, the chemicals added to soil and water change the magnetic field of the Earth, which is the mirror of the Earth. Whenever people add processed chemical products to the Earth, they thus also change the reflection of the Earth's magnetic field and ultimately, the magnetic currents.

The sun and its surrounding planets radiate onto the Earth, the dwelling planet of human beings. They permeate people and the Earth with their energies.

If the Earth's magnetic fields—as a whole, called the Earth's magnetic field—are no longer properly aligned with the irradiation of the sun and planets, because the mirrors, the magnetic fields, are opaque and partly torn, the Earth produces other values and also other animals, plants and forms again and again.

The magnetic fields have a variety of tasks. Among other things, they also initiate and influence the fertilization of the animals.

Just as they have an effect on the animal world, the so-called pests are also influenced by them: parasites and all the types of life that have emerged through the wrongful behavior of human beings. These, in particular, react to dissonances in the magnetic currents. This also applies to viruses and harmful bacteria.

The greater the potential of the negative forces grows, the greater the influence of dissonances in the magnetic currents on parasites, viruses and harmful bacteria, as well as on human beings and animals.

All other misdirections of the people, which are traced back to other wrongful behaviors of individuals and of the masses, also create causes in the soul. Sooner or later, these causes become effective in the body—or in the spheres of purification.

*More about the
significance of the nervous system—
the sounding board of the body—
Tension blocks the inflow of the life force*

It is precisely the world of people's thoughts that is the decisive complex that lends wings to them or shadows them, depending on how they feel, think, speak and act.

Thus, with their contrarieties, disharmonious people constantly influence their nervous system, which is the connecting network to the soul. They cramp the fine vital nerves, through which and along which flows the spirit power, the life, which wants to keep the body healthy and full of zest for life.

Due to the ignorance of many regarding the power of thoughts, the body withers away, despite external care; and the soul, the spiritual form in human beings, the book of life, shadows itself more and more. The soul records all the stirrings and inclinations in people, their feelings, thoughts and all processes in and on them.

If the nervous system is tense, then little life force accordingly flows into the body. The effect of this is that people create new causes, or that soul burdens break open, because they have thus come into zones of vibration that bring the soul burdens into effect.

Every cell of the body has a consciousness, a subconscious and a spirit consciousness. If the nervous system, the sounding board of the body, is tense, that is, disharmonious, then the eternal life force, the spirit consciousness, can supply the cells only minimally. As a result, negative forces vibrate into the cell's consciousness and subconscious and paralyze the activity of the cell tissue. This, in turn, results in illness, indisposition and blows of fate, which manifest themselves in many ways and become effective.

Therefore, at every moment, the nervous system registers the feelings, thoughts, words and actions of human beings—and also the resonances of the surroundings, both the positive and the negative vibrations. If the human beings are turned toward matter, then they will absorb from it the many different negative vibrations and become infected with them. The result is the further tension of the nervous system, from which, in turn, further indispositions, illnesses or blows of fate can result.

Without a healthy, balanced ratio between human beings, animals, plants and minerals, too, human beings cannot survive in the long run, because they are dependent on a balance between the forces of the animal, plant and mineral kingdoms.

The essence of life of the animals, plants and minerals is the cosmic forces, which, in unity with the forces of infinity, are in harmony. If people act against the kingdoms of animals and plants and against the mineral kingdom, they violate the law of unity, of harmony.

Those who violate the universal law of harmony cut themselves off from the direct stream, from God, from life.

Life is God, and God is unity.

Those who violate the universal law of unity consume ever more of their physical energies, which they then arduously want to maintain with food and stimulants. Suffering, illness, hardship and fate are the consequences. This, in turn, also implies that the animal and plant kingdoms will gradually die out and human beings will finally fall back to the Stone Age, in which they will have to arduously eke out their lives.

Whatever human beings deliberately destroy will, in the long run, die out on the external level. Those animals that bring with them a certain energy potential that contributes to the ecological balance will become fewer and fewer. The medicinal plants, which also contribute as radiation to the health of human beings and animals and to the wholeness of the entire atmosphere, are atomically contaminated and will die out. Stones will remain for the time being. What can human beings make from them? Very little.

This means that over the course of the times—after the Kingdom of Peace—the human race will die out, and the Earth will, in the further course of events, be led to eruption and expansion. Subsequent to this, an evolution will take place that leads to the fine-material.

That was just a brief overview to show what will happen in the coming millennia. The prophecy that I am giving here goes beyond the Kingdom of Peace on Earth.

Every animal has been given a certain task by God, which contributes to the good of all life. Every animal created by God has a positive task in the plan of creation.

Animals that live in the soil, the tiny animals and micro-organisms, are called the nature cleaners of the Earth. They aerate the earth, the soil, and prepare it for the incoming particles of the sun and moon. The fertile rays of Venus, Mars, Mercury, Saturn and other planets, as well, which the All-Spirit, God, has assigned to the Earth system, can then accomplish their positive task in and on the Earth: Via the elementary forces of fire, water, earth and air, they stimulate the growth of plants and minerals, thereby also contributing to the ecological balance.

If the ratio of these components is disturbed, then the ecological balance is not in the All-harmony. The result is that human beings come into disharmony. Many kinds of illnesses are then the effects of the causes mentioned above.

The pollution of water,
the source of life for the human body,
also leads to illness

In a drop of water there are countless living beings. This life force also contributes to the balance of life in the entire solar system. These countless life forms within the water drops contribute not only to the cleansing of the rivers, lakes and oceans, but in so doing, also to the welfare of the entire organism of the Earth. The organism of the human being, too, the human body, is cleansed by the water that contains the countless microorganisms designated for this task. I call these forms of life the nature cleaners of the physical body.

Humankind's relationship to nature and to water, the source of life, has been disturbed. The water of the Earth is not only given for cleansing and irrigating the soil, but also for the human body, its cells, blood and organs. The countless organisms in water, the microbes, contribute to the cleansing and detoxification of the intestines of both human beings and animals, and they build up the intestinal flora. Healing water is intended for all the components of the body.

Human beings consist primarily of water. They are dependent on the Earth and its wellsprings, water. If the wellsprings of the Earth, the water, are polluted, if they are no longer able to supply people with healthy, restorative substances, then people also fall ill. If the smallest creatures, the microbes, are destroyed in the water by chemicals, nuclear contamination and the like, then it is a lifeless liquid, which can still serve people for external cleansing, but no longer for restoring, strengthening and revitalizing the organs.

Thus, the causes leading to indisposition, illness and blows of fate are manifold.

Compared to infinity, the human body exists for only a moment or two. The soul, however, the ethereal body that dwells within the human shell, has eternal life.

The soul's task in its human body is to purify and cleanse itself, to delve into the holy laws and then to apply these to itself, to both soul and body, so that it may live on Earth in a right and lawful way.

As long as people do not live in peace with their neighbor, they are not in unity with the nature kingdoms either—and consequently, are not in unity with God, since God is all in all things.

Those who do not live in unity with God are in the law of cause and effect, in the causal law.

Whoever lives in this law will create new causes again and again—until they awaken in the Spirit and follow the laws of peace, harmony and love. The effects that follow the causes created by people are, as already revealed, illness, blows of fate, hardship and worry. People continue to live in this ever-revolving cycle until they recognize that they are cosmic beings, who belong to the divine unity, to the universal Spirit. If then people begin to allow this cosmic unity to grow in themselves, by recognizing the essence of life, the Spirit, and acknowledging it through the actualization of the laws, then they will become healthy—and through them, the Earth, rivers, lakes and oceans.

The causal law says: What you have done to the least of your brothers, you have done to Me, the Spirit in soul and person.—Figuratively speaking, this means: You have done this to yourself because you turn away from the Spirit of life, which is the life, from people who are your neighbors, from animals and plants, who are your second neighbors, and from the Earth with all its life forms. The result can be only illness, worry and hardship.

Live your life consciously!
Recognize the cause in time,
by monitoring your thoughts,
before it comes into effect

Once again, I want to make My human children aware of the reasons for the development of all illness:

Whatever causes people sow, they will reap—unless they repent of the causes in time; namely then, while they are still active in the consciousness or as a memory in the subconscious, or when they rise up and become effective as thoughts that do not correspond to My eternal law.

To recognize the newly created causes in time, it is necessary to monitor one's own feelings, thoughts, words and actions.

190

Every thought, both positive and negative, seeks to become effective. Every thought is energy and seeks a channel to express what has been placed into it. The more often one and the same thought is thought, the more intense is its effect.

Thoughts, words, and actions are seeds that fall into the aura, into the person, and then into the soul. If they are not recognized in time, they begin to germinate and sprout, bringing forth fruits of their own kind.

If they are not recognized in time, they go where large energy fields are active that radiate in a like or similar way as the thought of the sender. That is, they go to the "realm of thought" and there, they call up similar kinds of thoughts. The thoughts then band together into an energy complex and then return to the sender. They influence the sender and endeavor to cause whatever it was that the sender may have feared.

The stronger this returning energy complex is, the more intense its influence on person and soul. On arrival, the energy complex finds correspondences or memories in the soul, because the emitted thoughts correspond to either the memories or the correspondences of the sender. The energy complex also has an influence on the soul and may awaken further recollections or correspondences there, causing them to become effective.

If memories are awakened, these may also be of a positive kind. With awakened recollections of experiences or suffering, it may, for instance, be possible to help a second or third person now suffering the same or similar things. All of infinity consists of selfless service, because God is love. Therefore, selfless help is manifold. A person asking for help will receive help.

Animals and even plants can emit sensations that ask people for help. People who have a positive connection to the nature kingdoms will, if possible, be attracted by a suffering animal's surge of sensations or by groups of downtrodden plants and trees that need help. For the Spirit is at work over everything and in all things. The guardian spirits, given as help and support to people, also serve, help, and guide; the nature beings are likewise active in their own way.

Everything is vibration.

Like vibrations try to communicate with each other; unlike ones repel each other. This is the spiritual law of attraction and repulsion.

But memories can again become correspondences. Memories that were once burdens, but which have been atoned, that is, expiated, and merely evoke in people things and occurrences without emotions may, nevertheless, turn into correspondences again, if they give in to the waves of negative thoughts and let their life run its course without monitoring or controlling it.

At first, the waves of negative thoughts gently touch the memories present in them, that is, what they have already expiated and paid off. If they are not alert and start pondering about past events, they revive the memories. In this way, these may again become correspondences, depending on the content of the thoughts and their intensity.

This can happen as follows: People remember an event and think about it for a long time. They let the past flare up once again. In the process, a small negative aspect finds its way into their otherwise positive world of thoughts: a temporary agitation arises, that is, a few negative thoughts. These are strengthened by the vibrating negative thought waves and create their corresponding causes. In this way, a memory can become a new correspondence, a cause.

Over the course of time, this correspondence in the soul can also become effective in the body of the person concerned. This may happen as follows: by pondering, a person falls into zones of vibration in which pathogens are active. These now begin to have their effect and either evoke an indisposition or trigger further consequences or illness, depending on what's there.

Because of the indisposition, an appointment may, for instance, not be kept or even forgotten. This may perhaps cost the person concerned a lot of money or have other consequences. From the cause, "uncontrolled thought," which awakened a memory that brought further un-controlled thoughts, a chain of effects developed.

An anxious person may, for example, emit thoughts of worry. They come in part from a correspondence in the soul. They are burdens that initially come up only sporadically and are preparing to flow out of the soul. These thoughts go through the same process as revealed above: They move toward large energy complexes where they call up like forces. These combine and move from the realm of thoughts back to the sender. Depending on how often the person has thought and still thinks the same or like thoughts, they then gradually settle in the aura and start exerting their influence—from without to within—on the person as well as on the soul. Whatever the person was afraid of now becomes reality.

Often there is only a small correspondence in the soul or in the subconscious, a sphere of vibration that might have been transformed through positive thinking, without the person ever having to feel its effect physically. But since the person concerned allowed thoughts to chase through the brain without being monitored, the person is now chased by what has been intensified with thoughts. The small correspondence, a minor burden or even an occurrence long-since forgotten lying in the subconscious, now grows stronger and leads to effects because it was wrongly and frequently thought about.

If people often think of an illness, if they are afraid of it, then they attract the same or like thing. If they continually talk about their illness and indisposition, they reinforce them in the body—as well as in the soul.

Feelings of hatred, envy, hostility and revenge also lead to illness, suffering and blows of fate. The cause is always a wrong way of feeling, thinking, speaking and acting. The effect takes place either in or on the body, or else a blow of fate occurs in the immediate surroundings of the person concerned. Wrongful behavior is therefore the cause. The person obstructs the eternal, harmonious forces, the law of love and of peace.

If within a family there is illness, hardship, worry, grief, dissension, quarrelling, hatred, envy, hostility and blows of fate, causes always lie behind these. The cause always falls back on those concerned. They have to bear the cause as an effect. As revealed, it develops in or on them, or in their immediate surroundings.

Therefore, whatever people sow they will also reap, both the positive, all that is good, as well as the unlawful, all that is negative, unless they recognize, repent and clear it up in time.

Therefore, O human being, live your life consciously!

Each day wants to tell you what you should clear up on this particular day as well as what you may delight in with all your heart.

Every action is followed by a reaction.
The action first occurs in the brain, in feeling and thought. The reaction occurs in the nervous system and then in the cells, organs, muscles, glands and hormones, that is, in the entire organism. And as things develop further, the actions and reactions in the body have their effect on the soul, too.

Thoughts also stimulate the senses. The senses, in turn, have an effect on the nervous system and on the consciousness of the cells and organs.

Every cell is life and, as stated, has three aspects of consciousness: the spirit consciousness, the subconscious and the consciousness. Each cell belongs to a cell formation, which, in turn, has a spirit consciousness, a subconscious and a consciousness.

If the cell tissue has a high frequency of vibration because a lot of spirit power flows into the body via the soul, it repels negative energies. It protects itself by giving corresponding signals that are received by an alert person who then heeds them in thought and action.

The organism is always a mirror of what people once thought into their soul and into their organism—and of how and what they think today.

If a person thinks and lives positively, the cell tissue orients itself to a higher life and absorbs the higher forces. But it repels the higher forces, if it is negatively polarized. This is why a lengthy preparation is often needed for both body and soul before My helping and healing forces can make a breakthrough.

Every organ is vibration that shows its own particular color. The frequency and the color of its radiation indicate whether the organ is healthy or sick.

Vibration and radiation of color together form a tone. Thus, every organ has a tone. The tone, also called sound, corresponds to the condition of the organ. Everything the soul stores, whether beautiful, good, noble and pure, or ugly, burdened and dark, all these are tones, and thus, sounds. These energies, which are melodies, flow into the body via the consciousness centers and cause the organs, in turn, to vibrate and sound out.

Thus, everyone is a "body of sound," an orchestra, according to their burden, to their way of thinking, speaking and acting. Just as they think, speak and act, so do they radiate and sound. This shapes their whole behavior. Their entire external appearance is an expression of their burden and the "melody of their thoughts."

The whole universe is sound; it is melody, color and form, for even the fine-material forms are "radiation effects," since they are spiritual bodies that can be penetrated.

If an organ is sick, it emits dissonances in color and tone. These dissonances emanate from the consciousness and subconscious of the organ.

Therefore, as long as the consciousness and subconscious of an organ are burdened and emit signals of illness, the organ's spirit consciousness cannot become fully effective. This means that the Spirit, the Inner Physician and Healer, cannot become fully active in order to give life force and health to the soul and person. Both aspects of consciousness, the consciousness and the subconscious of the cells, dominate and block the help from the Spirit with the spirit consciousness of the cell—according to its burden, its color and its sound.

Holistic therapy

Thus, people who want to attain the healing that comes from the soul, from the Spirit—that is, who are not merely intent on the healing of the body and leaving the burdens in the soul—should endeavor to change their way of thinking. Instead of negative thoughts, such as thoughts of hatred, envy, fear, worry and despair, they should think thoughts of peace, hope, confidence, health, friendship and love.

They can also take measures to restore the body through knowledgeable physicians who work in accordance with the laws of life. To achieve in-depth healing, it is important that the physician soothe the nervous system and engage in counseling sessions with the patients, during which the patients recognize their difficulties and then strive to gradually overcome them. In this way, the consciousness and subconscious of the organs, that is, of the cells, can calm down. The person gradually attains harmony, so that the body can prepare for the self-healing that comes through the Spirit.

Knowing physicians strive to relax the patient's nerves. They should lead purposeful counseling sessions so that the patients may recognize their mental state and make an effort to recognize their all-too-human thoughts and impulses as the causes of the suffering.

The physicians should also endeavor to help those seeking healing to overcome their disturbing thoughts, inclinations and stirrings that harm the organism. Furthermore, they strive to support the organism to the point where the patients can develop positive energies, thus contributing to stimulating their organism for self-healing through the Spirit.

In counseling sessions with the physicians and by means of spiritual conversations that lead to self-recognition, tensions and chains of thought are released from the layers of the consciousness and the subconscious, provided the person seeking healing is willing to accept and cooperate.

Through self-recognition and by surrendering to Me what they have recognized, the patients become quieter. They gradually find their way to both themselves and the harmony they sought. This then makes it possible for the spirit consciousness of the affected organ to more intensely transmit the healing rays to the material substance, to the organ and the healthy organism.

This is holistic healing: The soul cleanses itself of its burden and the body is restored to health. Therefore, if the spirit consciousness, the consciousness and subconscious of the cells are in harmony, relief and healing may follow, through Me, the Inner Physician and Healer.

The healing of the body alone
should never be forced.
Complete healing takes place only
through the Spirit via the nervous system
and the spirit consciousness
of each cell

Because of a person's wrong attitude toward life, the spiritual life force in soul and body is reduced to the point where the organism has but little life energy. If the consciousness and subconscious of the cells are very burdened in vibration, in other words, if their vibration is low, the sick organ cannot be healed by the Spirit via the soul. Medications can accomplish some things on the body, but they cannot heal the soul.

It is not lawful for people to focus solely on their body, and to try to heal it by all means at their disposal. Whoever wants to force healing with medications—even if they think they have been successful since they have become well again—will merely numb the consciousness of the organ concerned and suppress the soul's burden, which may possibly have been on the point of flowing out. The new cause created by such or similar wrongful behavior has its effects, if not in this incarnation, then in one of the future ones.

Physician and patient should not want to force healing. Instead, the physician should rather try to harmonize and strengthen the nervous system and support the organs with natural medication, so that the Spirit—via the spirit consciousness of the affected organ—has the possibility of allowing the healing forces to flow more intensely into the organ and into other parts of the body.

Therefore, physicians should strive to bring the entire organism into a higher vibration so that the positive forces can become effective. They themselves, however, do not want to achieve the healing.

A healing without side effects can be brought about only through the Spirit. This is why the following holds true: The Spirit heals via the nervous system and the spirit consciousness of each cell. A complete healing can result only through the Spirit, God, via the nervous system and the spirit consciousness of each cell.

A person's harmonization and orientation toward healing by the Spirit, by God, is achieved with prayer, with positive thoughts affirming healing, with meditation and with harmonious movements, as well as with counseling sessions with the physicians, with spiritual conversations and by supporting the body with natural remedies, which should be prescribed and supervised by the physician.

*The premature disclosure of former
incarnations is unlawful.
In-depth healing through the
Inner Physician and Healer*

According to My eternal laws, it is inadmissible for unknowing physicians and psychotherapists, who have not delved into My eternal law and, therefore, have no knowledge of it, to influence the deep layers of the subconscious and the soul garments of patients. If, as a result of such measures, occurrences come to light that the patients cannot cope with, over which they ponder, get upset and develop feelings of guilt so that they are no longer able to cope with their life, then not only the patients create new causes in themselves, but the unknowing physician or psychotherapist burden themselves as well. Thus, both patient and therapist have created causes together.

If, for instance, through the practice of depth psychology, former incarnations are disclosed and the patient suffers from these disclosures, then an illness may possibly be the consequence. The depth psychologist prematurely addressed a cause lying in the soul, thereby causing it to become active at a point when the patient was not yet able to bear it. In this way, patient and psychologist both created causes, the effects of which they may have to expiate together in another incarnation, depending on the intensity of the cause. The patient is guilty because what is still concealed should not be exposed, and the psychologist may not intervene in unconscious processes that are not yet ready to become active.

Such negative occurrences, hidden in the subconscious, can often turn into positive energy if the person has, in this life, learned to think and live positively. Spiritually trained physicians and trained spiritual life counselors know this. For this reason, they do not intervene in the deep layers of the subconscious, but rather try to guide the patient to self-recognition.

This is the difference between spiritually unknowing physicians and psychologists and practicing physicians and psychologists who have been spiritually instructed as well as spiritually trained life counselors.

Those who rely on the Spirit and delve into and apply My law will also achieve healing through the Spirit. But those who rely solely on the flesh may possibly experience relief or healing, but only for a short while, because every illness bears within a deep cause; this means that the illness is not only in the body but often in the soul as well. Therefore, the one who relies on the Spirit will attain an in-depth healing that cannot be achieved by worldly psychotherapeutic methods. The latter is unlawful, anyway, because, as revealed above, events may be addressed that the patient is unable to cope with.

The time is ripe when, in many cases, the practicing physician in the world no longer knows how, and by what means, relief or healing can be offered to a patient. The time is ripe when more and more physicians look to the invisible, to what is effective behind matter. Many are searching and, sooner or later, they will realize that there is no other alternative than to rely on the Spirit, who is the Inner Physician and Healer of the soul and person.

The cooperation between Me, the universal Spirit, and physicians who unite divine knowledge and its implementation will be the ideal situation in the coming time. For in the polluted world, in many cases, only the Spirit can help the sick person. So, in the coming time, people will call more on the Inner Physician and Healer than on a doctor oriented solely to pharmacy.

Recommendations for those seeking healing:
Right thinking and praying—
Harmonious physical exercises—
Organ address—Meditation of tranquility—
Lawful nutrition—
Harmonious body rhythm—
Controlled speaking

The first steps that a person seeking healing should take are as follows:

Recognize that you live eternally.

Recognize that not only your body is ill but that, above all, your soul is shadowed, that is, burdened, and that it radiates the negative radiation into the physical garment, into your body—which then triggers the illness.

Once you are aware of this, then begin to pray in the right way. Pray to the One who has beheld and created you, to the universal Spirit, to God, your heavenly Father, who works through Me, Christ, your Redeemer. Pray with concentration. Strive to turn off all human thoughts and pray to within. Pray into your body and into your soul.

Endeavor to apply your prayers over and over again, that is, to live as you pray.

Endeavor to sin less and less.

Endeavor to no longer deprecate your neighbors and to no longer think or speak negatively about them. Find the positive and selfless aspects in them. Speak about them and be glad. This brings you inner integrity, inner calm and deep peace.

Then the negative mindset will gradually disappear. It is replaced by positive, constructive, vivifying thoughts of peace, harmony, happiness, love, health, trust, hope and strength.

So that such a transformation can take place, from unlawful thinking to a positive, constructive way of thinking and living, not only the physicians must do their part, but the patients as well. Those seeking healing have to be willing to turn their world of thoughts to the positive and, in this way, to reform their life. Patient and physician then enable Me, the Inner Physician and Healer, to become more effective.

Therefore, when you pray, O human being, let your human feelings and thoughts come to rest. Concentrate wholly on your prayer, for the right prayer is a dialogue with God, your Lord.

Harmonious, balanced physical exercises and the organ address—and, at the same time, a Christian healing, that is, healing by faith—and a meditation of tranquility will help you to find your way into the desired harmony so that I, the universal life, may heal your weakened organ and your entire body via the spirit consciousness.

If through harmonious, balanced exercises, through the organ address, through Christian healing and the meditation of tranquility, the desired harmony has been achieved, then those seeking healing should endeavor to remain in harmony so that the healing current is not interrupted. This means that they should think less and less about themselves and their illness, but rather increasingly encourage the positive, selfless forces which, particularly during the organ address, are directed to those seeking healing.

In such a balanced cosmic rhythm of soul and body, the harmonized people will also eat their food consciously. As a result of the harmonization of soul and body, seekers of healing will reduce the harmful substances they have preferred so far, for instance, large quantities of meat, nicotine and alcohol, and, provided they continue to raise their spiritual vibration, gradually abandon them. They will eat more lawful food, which the Earth gives in abundance.

By way of a conscious diet, that is, by partaking of the food as a gift from God, the spiritual potential of the food is also raised. These spiritual forces, too, will then flow to the consciously aligned person as additional strength for soul and body.

The All-harmony, God, heals. God is eternal harmony.

To attain the rhythm of All-harmony, of All-consciousness, the human beings should pay attention to their body rhythm.

People who want to achieve or maintain health should endeavor to move in a calm, balanced manner. However, this is possible only when the past has been cleared up and all-too-human aspirations and strivings no longer dominate them—when their words are selfless and their actions God-pleasing.

Only then, will they truly live. They will experience their day consciously and can also master it. Inner calm and harmony bring about concentration and achievement, a timely recognition of weaknesses and mistakes, at the same time providing the strength to master them in the right way. In this spiritual attitude, both soul and person remain in a higher body rhythm that enables a more intense inflow of the eternal power.

Mind your tongue, too, O human being. Speak only what is essential—and what you say should be noble, good and selfless, borne by understanding, good will, tolerance and love. Then you will remain in inner tranquility.

Much talking and many unessential words also draw from the physical energy and from the soul's "battery of life."

So never think or speak badly about your neighbor. For whatever you think or speak, whether it be positive or negative, comes back to you.

And in the case
of contagious diseases and cancer:
The cause is wrongful behavior

I repeat because it is essential for both soul and person:

All that is positive raises the vibration of soul and body. All that is negative transforms the vibration of soul and body down to spheres of vibration in which deep-lying thought vibrations are at work and which seek to influence the human being.

216

In the spheres of low vibration, viruses and harmful bacteria are also active. They can be absorbed by people who have slipped into these spheres of vibration. Even germs encapsulated in people may break open and become effective, if they transform their energy body down with base thinking, with hatred, quarrel and envy. Every illness is a negative vibration in the body.

If an illness is widespread, and therefore occurs frequently, it gradually becomes contagious. An illness that occurs ever more frequently is a negative thought complex that has been transformed down. This takes place as follows:

People think about the same disease over and over again, fear it and contribute to the fact that others, to whom they listen and whose opinions they accept, also have the same and similar thoughts about it. Triggered by the fear of this illness, a powerfully vibrating thought complex develops in the atmosphere. This energy complex has its effect on viruses and harmful bacteria and promotes their proliferation, often leading to mutations as well, so that they may even become carcinogens. Thus, it is possible that, as an example, cancer, the scourge of humanity, is transmitted by certain viruses and harmful bacteria, in other words, it is infectious.

At the same time, this thought complex has an effect again and again on those people who think the same or similar things. Thereby, the people are stimulated to think even more often and more intensely about what moved them at intervals, over and over again. In this way, too, the vibration of the human body is transformed down, thus reaching zones of vibration from where the very thing feared by the person is triggered.

The predispositions for this were in the soul. Yet they would not have become effective if these people had changed their world of thought in time, from the negative to the positive.

Such thought complexes also develop when, for instance, many similarly thinking people focus their thoughts on the production of chemicals, on processing the atom, on the production of weapons and many other things.

May humankind thus realize the great multiplicity of things that are triggered and brought forth through the effectiveness of these negative energies, which individuals would never be able to comprehend with their intellect. All these negative energies that are projected into the atmosphere then trigger, in turn, a chain of wrongdoings that, for example, leads to the pollution of the lakes, rivers and oceans or to the pollution of the atmosphere and of the Earth. Among these one must also include atomic radiation as well as the awakening of viruses and harmful bacteria and their transformation into germs that carry the risk of infection for an illness, which, as yet, has not been contagious, as, for instance, in the case of the "scourge of humankind."

Over the course of time, all these things together lead to the pollution of the atmosphere, the waters and the Earth. This, in turn, leads to the development of viruses.

I repeat: The scourge of humankind, too—namely, certain forms of cancer—has become contagious. Via the air these viruses get into the blood and have an effect on the body depending on their intensity. In many cases, they result in nodules which, if not recognized in time, spread and attack the entire organism, cell by cell.

Through the power of thought and environmental influences, what often merely lay dormant in the genes as a predisposition has become a virus or harmful bacteria. For example, there may be a predisposition for severe pneumonia in the genes. Because of the person's wrongful behavior, because of brooding, aimless, hateful and envious thoughts, the predisposition in the genes breaks open and attacks the body. The result is pneumonia: coughing, fatigue and the person is not as physically fit as before. Because of this fatigue, yet more unlawful thoughts attack, for example, thoughts of hatred and envy. The person broods over the past and forgets to develop positive thoughts.

Sick people may indeed take medicine. However, they get more and more entangled in their thoughts. They stir up the past more and more frequently, get annoyed with members of the family, are jealous of their colleague's position at work and quarrel and argue with their neighbor. In this way, they send out poisoning thoughts. Whatever they send out returns to them. All the negativity that falls back on them causes the vibration of their soul and body to fall deeper and deeper. In this way, they draw closer in vibration to those zones where contagious germs are found. Once they reach these zones, they will infect themselves; they become infected. They may, for example, absorb the viruses, containing, in germinal state, the predisposition for the illness that is a scourge for many people.

In this way, pneumonia, which might have been cured in a short time, through wrongful thinking now develops into cancer, which is called the scourge of humankind. And fear of a certain illness can trigger the very illness that is feared, providing the predispositions are present in the genes or in the soul. The cause is always a wrongful behavior. The results may be illness, indisposition and blows of fate.

*Positive thinking and living strengthens
the spirit power and can avert
many a thing in time*

If you do not want to create any new causes that lead to further negativity, such as illness and hardship, then endeavor to think and live positively. Therefore, never think or speak badly about your neighbor. What your neighbors have, what they say and what they do concerns only your Father in heaven and your neighbor, His child.

You can go to your neighbors and make things clear to them. However, you may not condemn them. For whatever you do to the least of your brothers, you have done to Me. Whenever you condemn your neighbors or speak badly about them, you reduce the spirit power, Me, the flowing and healing stream in you.

If you have spoken or acted badly toward your neighbors, then ask them for forgiveness.

If you obtain forgiveness, the eternal forces, the holy forces, will again become stronger in you.

Once you have obtained forgiveness, do not think about the incident anymore.

If your neighbors have wronged you, then pardon and forgive them.

Once you have forgiven, then let what has hitherto preoccupied you rest, for you have forgiven.

Those who have fulfilled the laws of asking for forgiveness and of forgiving find rest in themselves—and attain inner freedom and the greatness of their being.

Those who are free of hatred, envy, fear and of all unloving feelings and thoughts can attain soothing and healing in both soul and body.

A person with a positive attitude toward life enables Me, the Spirit, to nullify many an impending indisposition in time.

Therefore, recognize the cause and development of your illness and its consequences on yourself and your neighbor in all the details of your own life. The cause lies solely in you: How and what you feel, think and speak and the way you act is essential for your present and future life on Earth.

Two thousand years ago healing could be given to the simple, trusting people— Present-day people are externalized, disharmonious and full of doubts

At the present time, the so-called age of technology with its din and pleasure-seeking lifestyle of many people, the individual needs more than ever submersion, that is, meditation, to gain distance from the noisy world and the struggle to maintain a competitive edge over others.

Almost two thousand years ago, when I walked the Earth in a human garment, there were only the poor and the rich. Technology did not exist, and the din was still bearable. The simple, poor person lived more with nature and its forces.

224

Among the poor, the fight and effort to become rich by any means did not exist. To the poor, it seemed impossible to attain wealth. Only in the following epochs and particularly in the industrial age, did the middle class develop, bringing with it three categories of society: the poor, the middle class and the rich. And now, technology has made it possible for the middle class to achieve wealth as well. This goal brought with it the race and hunt for material goods. Those who are rich hoard more than ever—and the middle class strives to get rich. The poor have no chance of becoming rich. And that is why in many cases they content themselves with what they have. As long as they do not pursue the circumstances of the middle classes, they are more modest and, depending on the maturity of their souls, turn to higher ideals and values.

But almost two thousand years ago, the poor still lived more tranquilly and quietly; for there was no technology with its loud, discordant noises. Since for them, there was also no middle class standard, the poor were not so caught up in the desire for well-being and property. Therefore, the nervous system of the individual was more relaxed than that of today's human beings. For this reason, the spiritual forces could flow more strongly in many people. As a result, in those days, there were more healings through the Spirit of My Father.

At the time of the great healings through the Spirit of My Father, I, the Son of God, was myself incarnated, and lived in the high consciousness of the primordial power, that is, I was one with My Father in heaven. Part of My divine mission was to show the people what is possible through the Spirit. It rarely happened that rich people became healthy through the Spirit, God. Rather it was the poor, who trustingly and hopefully affirmed the divine. In their simplicity, they accepted what was given them—for instance, the healing power for soul and body. They became cured, healthy, through the Spirit in Me, Jesus.

In contrast to this, the people of today are very externalized. They doubt, ask questions and are often so burdened and disharmonious that they cannot put the laws of peace and love into practice so quickly. They speak a lot and think even more, instead of trustingly surrendering to the One, who knows all things, who is the health and strength.

People who put the eternal universal laws and the laws of nature into practice will have a youthful and supple body far into an advanced age on Earth. They are cosmic human beings, served by the forces of the All.

People who consciously live with nature, who orient their aspirations and strivings to the divine have a noble cast of mind. Their consciousness is expanded accordingly. An upright posture and a supple, youthful gait are often evidence of a person of the Spirit.

If people's behavior toward their fellow people and nature is positive, if they integrate everything that lives into their life, if they respect and cherish all creatures and nature, then their cast of mind will also be noble and kind.

People of the Spirit will also be strongly imbued by the Spirit, God. As a result, they develop a balanced rhythm of body and breathing, and the air in their body can be broken down into the necessary components for their organism. A further result is that the blood, the blood and lymph vessels, the muscles, organs, glands and hormones are sufficiently invigorated with healthy substances. Through this, conditions of fatigue and weakness diminish, and this means that they become more joyful.

Nature wants to be people's friend.

Those who keep the laws of nature and consciously go through nature as often as possible will supply their body with life-giving and life-supporting oxygen. The spiritual forces will flow into them more and more and will fortify and keep soul and body healthy.

In its make-up, the human body is like the Earth. Thus, it is a "nature body," and therefore needs the substances that are brought forth by nature.

If people's cast of mind is noble and pure, if their thoughts correspond to the divine order, in other words, if they are selfless, then they will also act selflessly toward the nature kingdoms and the elements of the Earth.

If individuals live in unity with all people, they also live in unity with nature. The result is a healthy, peaceful, happy and youthful life that reaches far into old age.

Human beings are just as dependent on air as they are on food. If they lack healthy air rich in oxygen, they will become ill even if their nutrition is good and natural.

For human beings to stay or become healthy, the proper interaction of all forces in them is necessary: They need healthy air, the right kind of nutrition, sun and rain. They need the Earth to bring forth the produce for their nourishment and healthy water to refresh their cell structure and revive their entire organism.

Those who disturb the harmonious course of the cosmic energies in themselves and on and in the Earth will be disturbed themselves. They will have to bear illness, suffering and worries, until they are one with the cosmic life.

Whoever causes suffering to people or to nature has to suffer this themselves. That is the law of sowing and reaping.

Oxygen is life.
The nature body of a human
being needs fresh air, movement,
a change of milieu
and the right kind of food

Healing via the nervous system is a fundamental aspect, which I want to make known to all people.

If the nervous system is shattered, no matter by what cause, then illness will occur where the organs are already weakened.

230

Natural oxygen and pure air contribute considerably to the relaxation and detoxification of the nerves.

Healthy air rich in oxygen carries life-awakening particles that the body absorbs not only by way of breathing, but also via the cells of the skin. Oxygen-rich air invigorates the whole person and even raises the body's vibration. A harmonious walk during which oxygen-rich air is absorbed calmly and without hectic breathing will even bring about the abatement of burdening thoughts of illness and worry.

If the cells have enough fresh air from nature, it often happens that the consciousness and subconscious of the cell tissues become calmer. The person is then able to gain distance from the usual thought patterns and problems. Through this, the cells are built up. When both material aspects of the cell, the consciousness and subconscious, have grown quieter, I, the spirit power, the Spirit, the Inner Physician and Healer, can work more effectively both in soul and body.

For this reason, a change of milieu is often advisable.

The human being is a "nature body" and as such, should also live with nature. Many people close their windows and doors, overheat their rooms and lock out the health-promoting oxygen with its life-awakening particles.

I, the Inner Physician and Healer, advise you to let the air stream into your rooms during the day as well as in the night! Open the windows and doors as often as possible; let the forces of nature flow inside and inhale consciously and harmoniously.

Clothing should also be considered. One should dress according to the season, not too warmly and not too lightly, depending on the weather.

I also advise that the windows be opened at night, no matter what the weather is going to be like. Rain, wind and cold, too, are diverse sources of energy. In this way, much oxygen enters a person's body. And this revitalizes and renews the cells as well.

232

Cover the body with clothing appropriate for weather and season. It should not be too heavy. And wear appropriate nightclothes. If it is cold, cover your head with a woolen cloth.

If it is possible to sleep outside on warm spring and summer days, one should do so. Nature, too, the source of energy for the life of a human being, relieves illness and heals, since I, the Spirit, Am in all things.

A person who sleeps outside on warm spring and summer days lies, so to speak, in life's fountain of health. If it is possible for you to rest and sleep under conifers, which are great oxygen-carriers, then very soon you will be able to feel the invigoration of the body, providing that you co-operate with a positive attitude toward life, thus harmonizing your nervous system. For it is via the pathways of the nerves that the eternal Spirit heals the physical body.

Harmony brings health. You obtain it through a selfless, harmonious life.

People who suffer from nervous disorders, or from a so-called incurable disease, or from a form of paralysis should provide their body with natural oxygen by taking walks in the woods or with corresponding resting places, for instance, under fir trees.

To achieve holistic healing of soul and body, it is also advisable to occasionally choose a place to stay with lots of woods nearby. Again, let it be said here that the change of milieu and the change of thoughts are vitally necessary for recovering health.

If sufficient healthy oxygen is in the body, the natural remedies taken by the person will be more effective. In the body, they come in contact with the vitalizing oxygen, which then stimulates the natural remedies into more intense activity.

The life-carriers in oxygen even bring about a higher vibration of the human body, so that the entire organism becomes more receptive for the positive powers.

The combined action of positive, affirming thoughts and words, of light colors, forms and sounds, of oxygen and natural remedies stimulates the spirit consciousness of the organs to more intense activity. The nerves relax and the eternal power, the force of healing and life, flows more strongly through the soul and into the body. In addition to all these positive aspects, there is, as revealed, the change of milieu, which is important so as to gain distance from the daily routine, from all those vibrations at home that keep influencing a person seeking healing. In addition, those seeking healing need the right kind of diet, which they determine themselves based on the vibration of their body.

With the change of milieu, with the increase of oxygen in the body, with exercise, the organ address, with colors, forms, sounds and fragrances, they attain a higher vibration. This causes the sensory organs to react in a more subtle way, signalizing what nutritional substances the body needs, also in regard to food. A harmoniously balanced body rhythm, in other words, a harmonious body, communicates via the senses to the human mind what food it needs to stay or become healthy.

Everything is vibration. Thus, human beings are nothing but a vibrating complex, consisting of feelings and thought patterns. If they change their vibration, then their senses also react accordingly.

Human beings are a body of feelings and thoughts which, providing it is in harmony, perceives precisely what and how much food it needs, or which food it lacks or does not agree with it. Those seeking healing should not select any food they dislike or which they feel is not beneficial for them. On the basis of their feelings and physical perception, which goes by way of their senses, they should supply their organism with the food their body desires at the moment via its signals. However, beware of any fanaticism in this, too.

In the clinics or houses of health, those seeking healing should be offered the opportunity to prepare a little menu for themselves apart from the community meals, if their world of feelings and senses is contrary to the menu for the community. A harmonious body indicates—via feelings and sensations, but also via sensory perception—which food it needs and which substances the cells need, in order to be strengthened and built up.

As already revealed, the human body is a body of movement. Therefore, the human being should move about in fresh air as often as possible. Hectic movements and forced marches are not advantageous. These cause dissonances in the body. As already revealed, any long and intense exposure to direct solar radiation should be avoided, especially during the hot summer months. Walks taken in regions of abundant woods or waters, for instance, along the seacoast, result in the penetration of sun and oxygen particles via the breath and through the skin, which then stimulate the entire body to recover its health. Work done in a balanced way in the fields and gardens also prepares the body for the intake of oxygen and results in a raised vibration of the body.

Oxygen is life. But oxygen, too, can become effective in the body only when, as already revealed, the outlook on life is changed: Purposeful, God-filled, affirmative and selfless thoughts have to replace negative, aimless, hateful and envious thoughts.

All this together will then have a stimulating effect on both soul and body.

If the cell tissue receives too little oxygen, the heart and lungs may be damaged. The coronary arteries weaken, contract and narrow. The circulation decreases and the heart has to work harder.

If a person is constantly restless and hectic, a heart attack may result, because this constant restlessness and hectic pace lead to short, quick breathing. Through this, the heart valves can also be affected and, via the heart, the entire organism.

It is a lawful principle that those who do not live in and with nature weaken their organism.

But people who realize that their organism is a nature body will also live with nature and affirm the laws of nature and the forces of nature, which also bring healing and help.

It is not enough to call out today "Lord, help me" and tomorrow to doubt the help of the Spirit. A firm faith in Me, the eternal Spirit, and an unshakable affirmation of the positive energies bring relief from illness and healing from within.

How natural remedies work

Good physicians support the body with natural remedies and strive to harmonize the nervous system. They know that strongly modified natural remedies that have become pharmaceutical medicines have side effects.

Natural remedies as such are more beneficial to the entire organism than chemical preparations, unless they are applied in high potencies.

As soon as people become aware that everything is based on vibration, they will be able to understand My revelations correctly.

Side effects can occur in all areas of the organism. If, for instance, a medication to support the digestive system is thoughtlessly taken so that food is digested more quickly and easily, even this can have side effects, because the medicine can affect totally different organs, especially if the vibration of the digestive tract is not largely in accordance with the vibration of the medication taken.

Every action is followed by a reaction, even within the cell tissues, if a medicinal complex has an effect solely on the consciousness or subconscious of the cell tissue. The result can be a high fever, chills, or even worse complications. Even symptoms of poisoning or circulatory insufficiency can be caused in this way. Therefore, people are called upon to support their organism, the nerves and organs, with natural remedies.

Good physicians, who have the healing of both soul and body of their patients at heart, begin to prepare the body with low-potency medication. They will increase the potency very gradually, depending on the course of the disease, but will refrain from administering high potencies.

The body is a living organism and, via the control center, the brain, signals what is beneficial or less beneficial for it. It also reacts when certain medications or foods do not correspond to its vibration. Those who live more with the Spirit, with their developed spirit consciousness, can precisely recognize the reactions of their body and also know what needs to be done.

I revealed that the human being should begin with low potencies. The potency of the naturopathic medicines should be similar to the vibration of the weak organ. Its vibration should be only slightly higher than the vibration of the weak organ.

If this procedure is followed, the consciousness of the corresponding cell tissue will be addressed first. Once the consciousness has calmed down and become attuned, the person will feel better because the pain may have abated. Thus, the potency of the naturopathic medicine can be increased. It then has a calming and fortifying effect on the subconscious of the cell tissue.

Once both the consciousness and subconscious of the cell tissue have been largely harmonized, the spirit consciousness of the cell tissue becomes more active: Life and healing forces are then increasingly called up by the spirit-cell-consciousness via the soul's core of being. In this way, a lawful course of events is initiated: Starting from the soul's core of being, the increased healing forces then flow through the soul and through the person's consciousness centers into the spirit consciousness of the cells and into the subconscious and consciousness of the prepared cell tissue.

Every sound consists of several components. For instance, a cry of fear or joy is composed of different sensations, stirrings, feelings and thoughts. It is therefore a complex consisting of various components.

Every sound is an action, be it disharmonious or harmonious. Every action already bears in itself a reaction. This means that every sound comes back as vibration to its author or to those persons who are in the sphere of vibration of the emitted energies. They are influenced by it or prompted to thought or action—depending on what goes out from the person who is on the same vibrational level as the sound emitted.

And sensation waves from animals that were and are tortured, mistreated or cruelly killed by human beings are vibrations that stay in the atmosphere and that come back, in turn, to those who torture and kill animals. The animals in the slaughterhouses also sense that they have to die a violent death. The fearful and agonizing sensations of these animals come back to the perpetrators.

Countless animals suffer agonizingly because they serve as laboratory animals. They are treated as objects, as though they had no world of feelings. All these and similar actions will trigger corresponding reactions.

The world of plants also leads a sensitive life. They, too, react both to positive and negative thoughts, words, sounds and actions. Those who meet plants, herbs and flowers—indeed, all of nature—in a loving and understanding way will receive nutritious and vital substances from them for the well-being of soul and body.

However, the one who violates the laws of nature, who tortures nature with chemicals, who tears out plants and throws them away, who cuts down trees and shrubs while filled with sap will hardly absorb from nature the substances that the body needs.

Plants react in very subtle ways. As revealed, their sensitive life reacts both to the positive and the negative. If a human being meets them in a lawful way, they develop both good and nourishing substances. If a person violates the life principles of unity and love, plants may also develop harmful substances. Just like an animal, all of nature registers the cast of mind of a person who roams through the woods, fields and meadows or who works in the fields, woods and gardens.

The vibrations emanating from animals, plants and even stones are of a positive origin, because the nature kingdoms cannot burden themselves.

However, if a person approaches the children of nature, the animals, plants and also the minerals in a negative way—be it with negative thoughts or actions or with environmental pollution and nuclear radiation—then nature reacts by changing its vibration. The spiritual radiation in the plant species and in the stones recedes. As a result, the plants develop other substances— no longer the natural substances that the body needs for a healthy life, but harmful substances, which, in the final analysis, human beings spread, poured out and still pour out. Chemicals and nuclear radiation, all things negative change the vital substances of plants, shrubs, trees, flowers and fruits in woods and fields, and of the grains, too. These harmful substances are also emitted by nature in the form of vibration. Since no energy is lost, it comes back to its author.

Mysterious illnesses—helplessness

Due to all these and other events, especially the person who affirms the world falls ill more and more. In the course of time, diseases have arisen that physicians are still puzzling about and making assumptions. However, they do not recognize the details of the causes of the symptoms. The causes of the appearance of an illness will be so varied and diverse in kind that, in many cases, the physicians will have no other recourse than to either admit they are at a loss, or to abandon all reason and irresponsibly prescribe doses of drugs and radiation, which not only give rise to increased physical discomfort but also result in mental agony and suffering.

Many physicians will change their way of thinking and apply holistic therapy, which, above all, is concerned with the soul and only then, the body.

However, holistic therapy can be applied only by those who have examined themselves and have changed their life, from human, intellectual thinking to spiritual knowledge and divine Wisdom.

So that all people may recognize themselves and reform their lives, I, the Spirit of life, give information, teachings and lessons. But everyone has to work on themselves. No one will have their unlawfulness taken from them. Everyone has to recognize their ego, their wrongdoing, and be willing to gradually discard it, that is, to no longer do the negativity. They must be willing to work with the law and not against it.

Physicians should endeavor to first strive to live and act according to the eternal law themselves, to then help and serve their neighbor in a lawful way.

In the near future, the doctors of this world will be powerless in the face of diseases never seen before in this form and will no longer know which medicine to prescribe. The clinics will also gradually fill up with mentally ill people.

Added to this, are the radioactively contaminated human bodies that will react in quite varied ways to the ever-increasing radioactive radiation. They will suffer accordingly.

During the course of these developments, many physicians will have to recognize their own ineptitude. In many cases, their medical skills will fail.

The illnesses of the coming times will, to a high degree, be caused by radiation damage resulting from the nuclear contamination of the air, the soil, the lakes, rivers and oceans. Even the food and everything that a person ingests—including medications and natural remedies—will, over the course of time, be radioactively contaminated.

Physical death strides along with a large entourage, touching all those who are dedicated only to the material, thereby becoming susceptible and receptive to negative vibrations such as nuclear radiation, viruses and harmful bacteria.

But to the same extent that negativity experiences its defeat, heaven opens up for the suffering creature.

God again sent messengers of light who incarnated and now serve the great Spirit, the Father in Me, the Christ, as instruments.

Into this world I also sent a being who, in the earthly garment, serves Me as a teaching prophetess and spiritual emissary. Through My instrument, I not only teach the laws in general, but I also give human beings indications and teaching instructions on how they can shape their lives to fulfill the cosmic law, the Absolute Law, so that they become and remain healthy.

Heaven has opened up and continues to open ever more, for all people and beings who are of good will and who are ready to actualize the eternal law of harmony, of peace and of love—in order to prepare themselves for the eternally harmonious cosmic forces, and to become healthy or stay healthy so that they may attain peace, selfless love and conscious knowledge. This path leads directly to the heart of God.

The inner shapes the outer and vice versa.
Harmony in terms of clothing

n Universal Life the following holds true: To the same extent that people are permeated by Me, they will also shine through their fellow people and brighten the world.

Those who are awakened in My Spirit change not only their habits. Their inner being radiates into the external appearance and fundamentally changes the person. The features of a spiritually awakened person become more noble. Their behavior is harmonious because their thoughts and feelings are in harmony.

The clothing of such a person is well balanced—also in the combination of colors. They know that the inner shapes the outer and that the outer has an effect on the inner. People of the Spirit avoid colorfully checkered fabrics because they know that as varied as a person's scintillating world of thoughts is, so will they dress.

Such colorfully shimmering and checkered fabrics have a disturbing effect on the aura, on the energy fields of both soul and human body. It is also advisable to avoid heavy fabrics and dark colors. These can negatively affect the disposition of a very sensitive person. They may perhaps make such a person emotionally disturbed and apathetic.

People who have weak nerves should not wear heavy and dark clothing. The weight of the fabric as well as dark and checkered fabrics stress the nervous system even more than it already is through environmental influences. Every external disharmony and dissonance have a disturbing effect on the person's soul and nervous system.

Therefore strive, O human being, to avoid these external contrasts as far as possible.

To counter all these opposing energies, people should, as far as it is still possible for them, change their way of living, from disharmony and being world-oriented toward a harmonious life, toward unity with God.

Those who follow My instructions will find the confirmation in themselves that I, the Spirit of life, Am the truth. Through My sacrifice on Golgotha, evolution as life-bringing salvation is granted to every soul and every human being. Through spiritual exercises, it is possible for both soul and human being to raise themselves from low vibrations to reach higher spheres, in which peace, harmony, health and strength are effective. Through a conscious alignment with the holy laws, over the course of its wayfaring, the soul becomes one with God, its Father.

God is everywhere. He is omnipresent. Therefore, it is possible for every human being to become one with the highest power. Those who strive daily more to attain the high goal of union with God will be served by the holy powers of infinity. They are no longer slaves to their passions and desires, slaves to their thoughts and feelings, but masters over their base nature.

Once people have found God, their soul has become the pure spirit body. They are then spiritual people, or subsequently, God-people: spirit of My Spirit.

*Why deeper insights into
the eternal laws can be revealed today*

In this world, all degrees of consciousness live side by side, or even together. Through this, many different frequency ranges exist.

Every vibration tries to influence the others more or less forcefully, depending on the degree and intensity of vibration. Higher forces of like vibration fortify and make one another fruitful. Unlike and low vibrations are not accepted by higher vibrations.

The universal law says that like attracts like and unlike repels unlike.

Because the degrees of consciousness differ greatly in this world, the understanding of the eternal truth also differs. Therefore, only as much can be revealed from the Spirit of God as people are able to understand in the era in which the spiritual wealth is given.

My word is meant only as guidance, and the explanations in My revelations are comprehen-

254

sible only to those who can immerse themselves in the word.

In this era of technology, I can reveal much more to My human children than in past times. Familiar with technology, people know about the law of attraction and repulsion. They work with vibrations and frequencies. They know about the various intensities of light and their effectiveness. They have insight into the atomic structure and know about gravitation.

Due to all this knowledge, I, the Spirit, can also convey to people deeper insights into the eternal laws of infinity—and into the law of cause and effect. People know that colors, forms and sounds are frequencies, that is, vibrations, and that everything vibrates and influences everything else. Moreover, the people have coined new terms for their discoveries, which I use to express Myself in the world and for My own, for My human children, because God does not have words—and therefore, instruments are necessary.

*My time has dawned—
the time of the Christ*

The time will come in which technology will also decline, because it was not applied lawfully and for the benefit of all human beings.

This great turn of time has already begun. People and souls are setting out. Those who have merged with the temporal will be grasped and moved by the temporal, and those who are with the Spirit, with God, will be merged with the primordial power. In this way, light and shadow will collide with one another more and more.

In the spheres of church, economy and science, the light is battling the darkness. Often it still seems as if the darkness would start its triumphal procession against Me, the Christ, and put Me, the Spirit, in My place. However, this is only seemingly so—not in reality.

The time has come in which I, the Christ, will emerge victorious. Despite battles, war, devastation, nuclear contamination and everything that afflicts the Earth and humankind, I remain the victor—for I Am the light of the world.

A deep spiritual foreboding grips many people who are in a struggle with themselves, with their base nature. They feel that something great is imminent and will come to pass, for a New Era, the era of the Spirit, is bursting forth from the negativity and will renew the Earth and the world.

The forces of infinity enter battle with the opposing forces.

For many people there will be a New Era, the era of a true humanity.

I, Christ, have initiated the New Era and My light radiates ever more intensely into the world and into the hearts of those who love Me. Through them and with them, I will grasp all those who are still oriented to the world; for all shall find their way home to the heart of their and My Father.

During the time of the increasing light of Christ, many sick people will receive help. The oppressed will find freedom and the enslaved will find the path to liberation.

My time has dawned, the time of the Christ.

I work through My own. Help and salvation come to those who suffer illness, hardship and hunger. Those who have been blinded will recognize their illusions and many will find their way to Me, the Savior of souls and the founder of a true humanity.

Come to Me, all you who are weary and heavy-laden! According to your faith, I will serve, help and give to you. Into the darkness of night help will thus come, the light of the world, I, the Christ.

I will free the enslaved souls and the frightened people.

The Earth will be transformed by the primordial power, just as the soul will be transformed by Me, the Christ. I make all things new. I bring everything into evolution, toward the Father, the light.

*A spiritual revolution will introduce
the true humanity. Let the one carry
the burden of the other—Pray and work—
Give and receive. The right help for those who
suffer need—A genuine missionary work*

The revolution in soul and person comes before this: They have to realize that the material thought up by people passes away, and the spiritual rises, it will indeed be visible through people of the New Era.

If, during the past two thousand years, souls and people had striven for the spiritual evolution, the expansion of the Earth's crust that leads to the bursting apart of matter would not have had to take place following the Kingdom of Peace.

The reverence for God demands that those who truly love God keep the eternal laws.

The bread of the spirit is the life of the body. For this reason, the law for all people striving toward God is: Let the one carry the burden of the other.

However, this does not mean that these may become a burden to the other because they are unwilling to work and earn their bread.

A just person helps the one who is on the path of justice. However, those who merely want to receive, and not accept any spiritual teachings and instructions in order to actualize the law of "pray and work," must go on suffering deprivation until they understand that they, too, are called upon to actualize the law of love and unity, which says: Let the one carry the burden of the other—let the one help the other. This means to support your neighbor by giving bread and clothing to the hungry. But be mindful that they keep the law of "pray and work." Support them, but at the same time, give them the possibility to work in the right way.

Today people may be rich because they have earned this harvest in a former life. But at the same time, they are called upon not to increase or hoard their wealth for themselves but to share it and give to those who truly are in need—not just externally but also in need of inner spirituality—insofar as they are willing to fulfill the law of "pray and work."

Every rich person in this world is merely a steward of wealth. Therefore, with their fortune, the rich should serve the common good. If, however, the rich remain externally wealthy because they hoard their wealth and consider it their own property, then they are poor in their inner being.

So that they may become rich in their inner being, they will have to become poorer, or even poor, in their next life—depending on how the soul that was once rich in its earthly garment thought and lived.

People who live in prosperity should serve the poor, both those who live among them in loneliness and poverty and those brothers and sisters who live in deprivation in the developing countries. This does not mean, however, that they should share only earthly bread. Both spiritual and physical bread must be offered in the right measure. This occurs through spiritual teachings and through the actualization of the law "pray and work."

Right prayer is a selfless, conscious work in accord with the eternal law. Whoever does not pray rightfully, that is, who does not live, think and work selflessly, will also have nothing to eat in the future. Those who do not work selflessly will have no bread in the future either. The law of sowing and reaping brings everything to light.

The law "pray and work" also demands that people nourish themselves according to the law of nature, and that their thoughts are selfless and their actions serve the common good. In this way, both soul and person become healthy.

Missionaries of the various religions travel around many countries in which people are starving. They carry out their activity in many places. For the most part, it consists of biblical preaching and of earthly gifts.

I ask: Of what use to the unknowing, shadowed souls and the sick bodies are the pious words of the Bible and the medications for relieving external suffering? Many of these needy and starving people lack the inner nourishment, the spiritual bread. This means that they lack the right attitude toward life. To motivate the human beings who live in hardship and hunger and are marked by their fate to strive for true insight and repentance, not only pious words and earthly bread and medications are needed.

A human being needs far more: Sick, starving and suffering people may well have to be built up physically first—but at the same time, they have to be given an understanding of the law "pray and work." They must be offered the opportunity to work.

Spiritual people are faithful workers in the vineyard of their Lord.

Those who work will also receive their reward.

And those who work rightfully and, at the same time, ennoble their being will achieve spiritual metamorphosis. The caterpillar, the downtrodden and oppressed person, will become a butterfly, a person of the Spirit.

People of the Spirit know the law "pray and work." They also apply it in the right way.

It is written: With the work of your hands or "with the sweat of your brow you shall earn your bread." This statement applies to all people who have not learned how to work rightfully and, therefore, are not an example for their fellow people and for all the people in the developing countries. To work rightfully means to give first and then receive.

However, you shall not give in order to receive. Give and serve selflessly. This is why it is not lawful to give only bread to people suffering great need in the developing countries, without encouraging them to work in the right way.

Those who merely take and do not learn to give, which is an aspect of all work, remain one-sided in their orientation. People who are one-sided in their orientation are of the opinion that only their neighbor should give, while they themselves can only receive since they possess nothing.

Therefore, the one who takes should also learn to give. The law of "pray and work" contains both giving and receiving.

Over the course of time, the attitude that only a certain category of people should give causes a lethargic attitude in those who only take. Such an attitude can lead only to complications, since it does not correspond to the universal law. Such an attitude can lead only to further impoverishment and to yet greater chaos, since a counterbalance is lacking: pray and work, give and receive.

When the scales of justice, which have one weighing pan for what is given and another for what is received, are burdened on one side only, then sooner or later this means hardship, illness and lingering infirmity.

It is a life task over generations to give the people who think only of taking, especially in the impoverished, underdeveloped countries, an understanding of the law "pray and work."

This reformation from taking to the right proportion of giving and receiving can be brought about only by Christians who recognize in their inner being the eternal laws and also practice them. Only such people can build up one-sided oriented souls and human beings.

Although many missionaries are in service, only few render a just service in humility and selflessness, according to the law of love and freedom. Readings from the Bible alone do not induce a person to fulfill the law "pray and work." People with a one-sided orientation have to be taught and guided in accordance with the eternal law.

Hunger and need are outer signs of inner impoverishment. However, this does not mean that such people should remain in this condition. It is written: Let the one carry the burden of the other. Thus, Christians are called upon to stand by their poor brothers and sisters, to teach them the law "pray and work," to be living examples to them and to instruct them so that the law may be fulfilled: Let the one carry the burden of the other and let the one stand by the other in a lawful way.

Since in the developing countries the law of "pray and work" is not, or only partly, applied, there is great discontentment among the poorest of the poor. Waves of envy, enmity and accusation toward the neighbor who lives in affluence go out from there to the wealthy countries. These forces of envy, of enmity, of hatred and of accusation particularly influence those who do have the means and possibilities to assist the poorest of the poor in the right way, to support them and to teach them what is meant by: The one who works will have bread, and the one who lives according to the eternal laws will never starve and live in want.

This genuine missionary work has been neglected on a broad basis. This is why My call still applies today: Go out, teach and baptize. With the word "baptism," I mean baptism in the Spirit. Once someone has largely actualized the eternal laws, the Spirit permeates them, and they have again become spirit of My Spirit.

At the present time, I am again teaching those who love Me and who strive to dedicate their life to Me.

Guided by the eternal Spirit, people of the New Era will fulfill what is lawful: to teach even the poorest of the poor the law of "pray and work" and instruct them how this has to be done in daily life, in order to have physical and spiritual bread.

However, as has occurred so often in the past two thousand years, they are again being despised by many sham Christians who speak evil of them, because they think and live differently than the externalized Christians. Especially in the name of a state or ecclesiastical authority, those who lived and taught the true Christianity of neighborly love and mercy and wanted to carry it into all the world were always mistreated and tortured in My name. The times of cruel acts of violence are not yet completely over.

But despite all things vile, the new human being who fulfills the laws of life is now awakening, while the worldly person gradually wastes away, weakened by sensuality, illness, grief and radioactive contamination.

The New Era will be introduced with the cleansing of the Earth, since it is polluted and radioactively contaminated throughout all regions.

It will all be new.

The Earth's furnaces are the oceans, which are heating up through nuclear radiation. The Earth is the hotplate of the oceans. It will bring many things to boiling. Volcanic activity will increase, and the polar caps will melt. Radioactivity will increase. Not even the smallest of herbs will not be contaminated. The axis of the Earth will change, and the heated oceans will cleanse the Earth. Furthermore, there will be a change in the planetary constellations. Planets will also help bring about the cleansing of the Earth through their radiation.

A new heaven and a new Earth will emerge.

People of the Spirit will inhabit the new Earth.

People of the Spirit learn to help people in the right way, using the simplest of means, yet equipped with the most valuable power: with the all-sustaining Spirit of Love and Wisdom.

The time will come when the poor, too, will be granted what restores them spiritually and physically: a life in the Spirit that also gives physical bread.

The new human being will come who lives in Me, who teaches and through whom I heal, I, Christ, the life.

I, the Spirit, bring the Kingdom of God, the Kingdom of Peace, to all those who are of good will.

God's love comes to this Earth through My own. May the one who can grasp it, grasp it.

I Am come again to help and to heal, to serve My own.

The fire of the spiritual revolution is burning. I, Christ, have ignited it.

Again, it is said: Go out, teach and baptize! May the one who has ears, hear.

Thus, the causes created by humankind are manifold, as manifold as the effects, the illness, suffering, worry and hardship.

The causes were sown. What has been sown is now coming into being and has its effects in matter.

That is why I call this revelation: "Cause and Development of All Illness."

Many who today call themselves Christians, who live in affluence and work against My word, will, through the linkage between causes and effects, be plagued by hunger and pestilence in the next incarnations, because today they are pouring poison into the germinating true Christian life.

The law of "like attracts like" means that a burdened soul can incarnate only in a body whose hereditary disposition corresponds to the burden of the incarnating soul.

Thus, those who today want to trample on the germinating true Christianity and those who, in the face of those who live in poverty, unhesitatingly continue to splurge in prosperity will one day be called to account for it. Those who today do not live and teach the law of "pray and work" in the right way, and do not include the poorest of the poor, will one day suffer for their attitude.

Many a one believes that all those who live in sin and are burdened, who have to starve and be destitute, would have to expiate through this and that therefore no help would be needed for them. This attitude is in conflict with the commandment of neighborly love. If there are incarnated souls bearing a very heavy burden in the developing countries, this by no means implies that they simply have to expiate what they once caused.

According to the law of neighborly love, those who are not living in poverty and infirmity should come to their aid. However, this help should go beyond earthly food and pharmaceutical products—and beyond the word of the Bible.

Only the word that is lived is powerful. The word is the law. "Missionaries" must first put it into practice themselves. If the eternal law is actualized, then there is no longer need for literal readings. Nor is there any need for pious books.

It is the lived word, which is not only spoken freely but is also put into action in the right way.

God has no secrets

In the school that leads to the inner truth, people learn about the deep eternal laws. They are instructed in such a way that they can understand the eternal laws of God correctly and are able to apply them to themselves and then in the world. This is why I also give insight into the inner processes of genes and hereditary dispositions with regard to an incarnating and incarnated soul.

The new person, in whom the eternal truth begins to sprout, who blossoms in the fulfillment of the Sermon on the Mount, is not a blind one who believes that God lets no one see into the secrets!

God has no secrets from people unless they have secrets from God. This means that if people close themselves off from the divine stream, then they do not know the laws. Those who do not know the laws are blind to the truth. Only the spiritually blind will say that God lets no one see into the secrets.

If God, our eternal Father, had secrets from His children—if He had to hide thoughts of creation and lawful processes from them—then God would be imperfect just as the human being is imperfect.

Those who live in My following fulfill the eternal laws. I came into this world to teach and live the laws—not just to talk about them!

Those who follow Me are called upon to do likewise. Then the spiritual eye will open: The human being beholds the Being and not just the appearance. The secret is aired because the person has become divine. The veils have fallen; the mists of the human ego have dissolved. The person clearly beholds the truth.

The spiritual laws in procreation

Thoughts are powers. They can have an effect on the genes of the woman as well as on the genes of the man, depending on the nature of the thought and the predispositions in the genes.

The predispositions in the genes are decisive for the nascent gender. It is determined by both the woman and the man, provided they are in the law of cause and effect. In both genders, in the man and in the woman, the predispositions for the feminine and the masculine are found. The partners determine the gender of the child on the basis of their "internal clock," which is based on the law of cause and effect.

If the energy potential of both partners is mostly in agreement at the time of conception, then primarily a female principle is created—as long as the agreement does not change after a few days. If the woman dominates in terms of energy, then emerges—also under the prerequisite that the gradient of energy does not change—a male being.

Therefore, if the woman's energy potential is stronger than that of the man, then the male aspects in the woman will begin to vibrate more. Consequently, the woman is superior to the man in terms of energy. Through this, predominantly male aspects are stimulated in the egg that is being fertilized. Consequently, a male being begins to grow in the womb of the mother.

In the egg that is about to be fertilized, a powerful control mechanism is at work that is kept in motion by the constellation of the planets—according to the burdens of the two partners. Through this lawfully controlled process, the egg that is being fertilized attracts the forces that are more intensely active in it. For the physical union of woman and man does not happen by chance, but is the effect of previous causes.

There is also the physical union of both partners through the Absolute Law. This takes place when both man and woman are no longer under the causal law, the law of sowing and reaping.

If the partners procreate a child on the level of the Absolute Law, then the sperm and the egg are without burden. They are not irradiated by the law of cause and effect but by the pure law.

Like attracts like. In such a case, a child is born that bears within high ideals and values: the life from the Spirit. It is in this sense that the procreation of Jesus of Nazareth should be seen, in whom I, Christ, incarnated.

Feelings, thoughts and words are forces. They can either rise from the soul, or they "come flying" from without, and are absorbed by soul and person—provided there is an existing correspondence, a predisposition.

Positive as well as negative sensations, thoughts, words and desires can—if they are moved again and again—have an influence on the genes according to their intensity.

This means that both the man and the woman have an influence on their own genes—and also on the egg that is about to be fertilized.

If the energy potential of nature begins to fluctuate, for instance, after wars or disasters, and there is a considerable lack of male or female principles, then the law of nature provides a balance:

Just as the moon in conjunction with the sun and other planets controls the tides and stimulates and regulates the mating of animals via the magnetic currents, in a similar way the radiation of the stars affects human beings more intensely via the magnetic currents, when the energy potential between man and woman is subject to significant fluctuations.

If, for instance, there is a lack of male beings, the moon will, in conjunction with the sun and the stars, stimulate the male aspects in the genes. The moon—in conjunction with the sun and those stars that at the time of conception have a special influence on the people with a corresponding degree of vibration—then gradually restores the male-female balance to the extent that it is sufficient according to the natural laws of attraction—also called polarity.

The balance of forces, including that between man and woman, is a part of the consonance of energies of this Earth and of the whole solar system.

Human beings are called to uphold the laws of infinity and to apply them to themselves and to the Earth. If this does not take place because human beings intervene in the harmony of forces, in the ecological balance, then their relationship to their environment—and to their neighbor—is also disturbed.

Therefore, O human being, be alert, because every moment in life bears within new, that is, other aspects in your thinking, feeling, wanting and acting that correspond to your soul burden and to your present way of life.

Joy and suffering, illness, health and well-being are determined exclusively by human beings themselves. People are the builders of their own destiny and their own lives.

At any given moment, all people are faced with the decision: for or against the eternal law. Their feelings, thoughts, words and deeds are their life; these are what the person is. With what the people are, they influence their surroundings— but also themselves, because what they sow they will reap, both positively and negatively.

Thus, a mother-to-be can, according to her thinking and living, also have an influence on the genes of her unborn child. If the life of the expectant mother is balanced and harmonious, if her feelings are noble and her thoughts good, if she lives consciously, that is, in the certainty of God's omnipotence that embraces everything—including her growing child—then it is possible that many things can still be changed in the genes, which, at the moment of procreation, might have hung as a sword of fate over the man, the woman and the unborn child. Whatever is changed in the genes of the mother can also be transformed in the approaching soul, insofar as this is good for the soul.

However, not only the woman but also the man has a great responsibility toward the unborn child. The man likewise plays a decisive role in determining which soul can incarnate. The man's positive, loving and tolerant attitude toward the woman is decisive. His attitude not only has a positive effect on the mother but also on the unborn child, and, over the course of time, on the entire family.

The law of cause and effect also influences the relationship among the genders, because it is possible that they develop a joint karma through wrongful thinking, feeling, wanting and living, through quarrel and strife, which will show its effects sooner or later. Such a joint karma can also have an effect on the growing embryo in the mother's womb, if similarities also lie in its genes.

As long as people are under the law of cause and effect, they can be influenced in many ways, both in a positive as well as a negative sense. In this respect, the man and woman can, already at the time of procreation, set the course for the approaching soul. According to the hereditary predisposition of both parents and according to their present living habits, which may tend towards the positive or the negative, a soul then incarnates. This is why all human beings are called upon to cleanse their soul and refine their body, so that further causes are not created.

So that human beings can mature and grow, they should first pay attention to their soul and then to their body. A healthy soul, that is, one that radiates with a high vibration and is free of major burdens, also has a healthy body.

The Spirit of life calls on human beings to raise themselves from their present sphere of vibration through a well-behaved life oriented to God, in order to reach higher, purer and more subtle vibrations.

As long as person and soul linger on the lowest level of vibration, that is, in the areas of earthly vibration, they will be affected by all the unlawful forces of pathogens that are effective in this area, in this vibrational zone. This applies to all souls and human beings whose vibrations are identical with the Earth's vibration—including the expectant mother and her child.

If, for instance, a mother-to-be contracts a pathogen that plagues her and perhaps confines her to her sickbed, the embryo may also suffer, depending on the type of germ and the intensity with which it shakes and afflicts the body.

Healthy food of high vibration also has an effect both in and on the human being, as well as on the child carried under the mother's heart.

I repeat: Everything is based on vibration.

Every continent, every country, every city, every town, place and house has its own vibration. For instance, people who inhabit a particular country are, in terms of their consciousness, a part of that country's vibration. Furthermore, the people who inhabit a country are individually brought together in cities, towns, places and homes, again according to their consciousness. Even the climate or the crops share the country's vibration. This is why people should mainly nourish themselves with the crops grown on the land of their native country or where they live for a prolonged period. Country, climate and natural products have largely the same vibration.

Since like attracts and reinforces like, people should also observe this principle to attain outer and inner harmony.

The fruits of perennial plants have more life force, since the plant is more closely connected to the cosmic rhythm. The mother-to-be, in particular, should bear this in mind. The high vibrations of fruits from perennial plants have a positive effect on the embryo, too. An apple, for instance, has vital substances that hardly any other fruit contains. In the various countries there are other fruits that have a high energy potential and that have an invigorating and strengthening effect on and in human beings, in the mother and in her unborn child.

If people live consciously at every moment, they will also absorb the precious, positive life forces at each and every moment—including the mother for her unborn child.

From the moment of conception, the embryo is dependent on the father and the mother— indirectly on the father via the mother, and directly on the mother.

Just as the positive as well as the negative energies reach the embryo via the mother, lawful or unlawful food also has its influence on the human being, on the expectant mother and the embryo.

The New Era, the era of the Spirit, will bring forth people of the Spirit who are healthier. Through this, their children, too, will be healthy and vigorous when they come into this world. The New Era will know less and less illness.

In all the repetitions, which are necessary for better understanding, I, your Redeemer, am endeavoring to shed light from many perspectives on all the processes and elements that affect human beings—both positively and negatively—so that the person can grasp My revelation in all its aspects and come to know the causes that bring about their effects.

The age of the Spirit leads many people who are striving for higher goals and values to the higher forces and soul vibrations of harmony and peace. Higher vibrations have a positive effect on people. They harmonize the organism and bring peace to their way of thinking and acting.

The higher the vibration of soul and body, the stronger the powers of resistance in their body. Those who are no longer mentally and physically under the influence of the radiation of the celestial bodies, that is, who have moved beyond the influence of the planets in terms of vibration—beyond the four astral planes—have a thoroughly illuminated and spiritualized soul and a correspondingly permeated body. Those who have risen above the sphere of influence of the planetary constellation are largely liberated from the law of cause and effect, the law of causality.

Spiritual development also includes the genes, so that negative hereditary factors are either eliminated or merely have a limited effect.

Nature gives manifold examples and similes for the development, the becoming, the growth and life of human beings and for their blows of fate and sorrows.

People are able to read the components of their own fate in natural phenomena.

An example of this:

In an earthquake, the epicenter, from where the quake has its origin, is shaken most strongly. People living in this vicinity can lose all their possessions. They may even be hit and hurt by their own collapsing house. Such a shock may even shatter their nervous system. For instance, one person may be hurt by a collapsing house, another one may suffer physical death, the next one may suffer a shock and yet another one gets off with a fright. In this, one can understand that this has something to do with the individual person's soul burden. According to their soul burden, people attract the negative forces that then have an influence on them, for instance, by way of collapsing buildings. The shadows of the soul are like magnets. They attract the same or like things from without.

Another example: When a volcano erupts, the areas directly at the foot of the volcano are flooded with lava, whereas more distant regions are only partly affected.

It is likewise in the life of individuals. If, for example, someone's vibrational level is at a greater distance from the vibrating complex of a pathogen, they will be only slightly infected and merely feel indisposed. But, if soul and body are close or even in the direct area of activity of the pathogen, these people will be more severely infected. According to their soul burden, they can become sick or even suffer. Decisive is always the type and intensity of the burden, which lies in the persons themselves.

In a positive sense, it is similar with the healing and life forces: The closer soul and person come to the primordial source, God, the healthier, the more harmonious and peaceful is the person. Once someone has drawn close to their divine origin, the healing and life forces will flow more strongly in them, and the cell tissues are aligned with the spirit power.

Therefore, O human being, learn to control your body. Curb your thoughts, refine your senses and you will move into more subtle spheres of vibration, into zones where the light, God, can work in you more intensely.

As long as people are at the mercy of their thoughts, they have no mastery over their senses. They are the passionate ones who simply create suffering again.

Those who want to stay or become healthy must put their thoughts in order, curb their speech and master their senses. Then they can be the master of their body. Once they are thus oriented to the divine, the spiritual forces consciously serve them in all situations of life. Those who live in God can move mountains in and around them. This means that their word has power and all that surrounds them will serve them.

Those who are in harmony with God, their Father, are also in accord with their body. This means that they will neither lament about their body nor complain about their condition. They will direct positive thoughts of healing and of peace into their whole body, to their organs, muscles, glands and hormones.

Those turned to God will not complain about an indisposition, but rather ask themselves what turned them away from their striving toward a life in unity with God. They will ascertain the cause of the disharmony. Then they will clear up what they have recognized about themselves, to again consciously strive toward the unity with God. The growing unity of spirit, soul and body results in health, strength and happiness.

Those who live in unity with God live consciously.

Those who live in the unity of spirit, soul and body are also able to successfully address their organs and their cells.

Those who are in harmony with God will be obeyed by all subordinate areas, the whole organism, for instance, the organs, glands and hormones.

Those who are in harmony with the divine also have a positive influence on medications, foodstuffs and beverages.

Through communication with the All-power, spiritually trained people are able to establish a spiritual communication with the individual organs of their body, since, as already revealed, every organ and every cell has a consciousness, subconscious and spirit consciousness.

When people are in harmony with God, the spirit power radiates more intensely throughout their soul and body. This means that the spirit consciousness of the cells is active and dominates the consciousness and subconscious of the cells. As a result, the cell tissues that are aligned with the Spirit immediately react to the highly vibrating thought waves that spiritually oriented people send to their body. Since the entire organism is one vibrating complex, in which each organ vibrates according to its permeability, each organ can also be addressed by the person.

Thoughts and words are forces that are absorbed by the cells and organs. An echo forms in the organism, in the cells. How people think, speak and act is how their body, the cell tissues, reacts.

The consciousness of the organs reacts both to a person's positive and negative impulses and to impulses from the immediate surroundings.

Those who have learned to master their thoughts and senses can also prepare their body for healing by the Spirit.

Recognize, O human being, from My manifold and repeated explanations, what the causes of all illnesses and occurrences are and in what way they develop.

Thus, consciously become one with the universal Spirit, with your soul and your body, with every organ.

Recognize your body as the instrument of your soul, as the vehicle of the spiritual body that dwells in you. Your thoughts, words and deeds and your attitude toward life are the fuel for your body.

Through technology, human beings have machines, vehicles, airplanes and much more. Should the vehicle or airplane transport you from one place to another or from one continent to another, the tank has to be filled with fuel and not with water. And the transmission system is filled with transmission oil and not with vegetable oil.

You know that the engine of your vehicle or airplane can work and perform properly only when it gets the proper fuel and oil.

Human beings are careful to supply their vehicles and airplanes, their machines and everything produced by technology with proper fuel and electricity.

However, they pay little attention to their soul and to the vehicle of their soul, the body.

The vehicle does not run and the airplane does not fly without the proper fuel—and a person's body does not function without the Spirit, God.

The human body is a nature body, of which all components or substances come from nature. This is why human beings should live with nature and recognize the motive power, the life, the Spirit, in all the forms of nature. Then they would soon become aware that I, the Spirit, Am closer to them than their arms and legs.

When people realize that they are a part of nature, they will also come to recognize themselves and understand the workings of the Spirit in matter.

Then they will also realize that they are not only body, but that in their body there is an indwelling spiritual body—and that the physical body is merely the vehicle of this spiritual body that dwells in them.

The soul has incarnated to expiate in the present incarnation its shadows or a part of its shadows, the burdens from previous incarnations. This is why it should be a commandment for people to keep their body healthy through healthy food that comes from nature, through pure thoughts and through a lawful life. Experience your body as the vehicle of your soul!

Become one with each organ by giving it the necessary nutrients found in nature: in the fruits of the fields and woods. Vivify both soul and body through positive thoughts, thus bringing about the unity with the Spirit.

The organs readily absorb the substances from nature if you, O human being, lead a positive and harmonious life.

People who are largely in harmony with their body and behave according to the laws of God in their daily lives are also able to interpret the warning impulses given by the organs. This sensitivity can be attained by every person, provided that they fulfill the universal laws, thus finding their way into unity with life.

Human being are children of the All. Once their soul is light-filled and their cast of mind pure, they are in communication with the cosmic forces.

Therefore, those who want to come into harmony with the forces of the Spirit have to overcome their base nature, their passions and human feelings. They have to break the fetters of hatred, envy and ambition, which hinder the divine power from serving and helping the human being.

If alert people consciously strive for the unity of soul, spirit and body, if they are free of compulsive thoughts, desires and expectations, and have attained spiritual maturity, they can learn from their own consciousness what they have to change in their life so that their body may gain strengthening, health and capability. If someone is spiritually awakened, it often makes more sense to engage in conversations about their way of life, their attitude and their behavior than to immediately turn to natural remedies, or even pharmaceutical products.

*A right way of thinking
and attitude toward life are
more important than medications.
A counter-example: the self-destructive
attitude of a patient*

Those who recognize their momentary situation and change their way of thinking are already today preparing for the time when there will be neither healthy medicinal herbs nor helpful medications.

Even natural remedies should not be taken lightly. In many cases, a healthy attitude toward life will prove to have a greater effect than natural remedies or even pharmaceutical products.

Recognize that thoughts are forces. They influence and control the body—even the desires and will of a person. The body is influenced according to the intensity of thoughts, whether positive or negative.

Every knowing person will strive to cleanse soul and body from negative feelings, thoughts and words—and to keep them pure. Healthy nutrition is a part of this. The effects on the body have, in turn, their effects on the soul. Just as people think, so are they—or will be.

Here is an example from which every person can learn, for themselves or for their family:

Today people are happy. They affirm life and are friendly to all their fellow people. They are in harmony with their environment. Their feelings are refined, their thoughts good. They are convinced that luck flows to them from all spheres of life and will smile upon them. In their family, everything is well-ordered and everyone seems to be in harmony. Their friends are one with them. Everything is fine. They are healthy; they also enjoy culinary pleasures, alcohol and tobacco. For them the world is full of sunshine.

One day they awaken from a restless sleep. They feel slightly indisposed. Their thoughts are gloomy even though the sun is shining. Their cheerfulness is gone. Worries and fears creep up on them. During the night they felt unwell. Certain processes become noticeable in their body that they cannot interpret and therefore make them thoughtful. They are depressed because they have heart pain, and their breathing is difficult. During the following day, dizziness, exhaustion and nausea set in. Their families are worried and their friends advise them to take this or that drug and to do this or that. They are advised to obtain medical advice. The physicians' diagnosis is cardiac insufficiency or a cardiac defect. They inform the patient of possible associated symptoms.

As a result of the diagnosis and information, those seeking help feel seriously ill and handicapped. For fear of possible consequences, they hardly dare to walk or breathe. They now observe every stirring and every pain in their body. "I am sick," they think and say.

What happens now to these people, once so full of joy, whose environment was nothing but sunshine and joy? Thoughtful and sad, they sit in a comfortable chair. Their surroundings, in which they live, are still bright and friendly. Yet they hardly notice them. Their mood is dreary. They are burdened with thoughts of worry and illness.

Their family members show concern about their illness. Nevertheless, they attend to their obligations and pursue sports and games. Their friends, too, attend to their usual obligations and pursue their pleasures. Their family and friends take them along, the so-called sick ones, to games and sports, but they —according to the physicians' diagnosis and their own doubts— can no longer practice these activities that they liked so much. They become resigned and feel more and more sorry for themselves. The result is that they stay away from all entertainment and pleasures.

They do not even attend to their usual activities at work or at home, since the physicians advised them to rest. Their nutrition, too, their eating and drinking habits, had to be completely changed from one day to the next. Everything they were fond of, what once used to fill them with joy of living and make them happy, they can now experience only through others, as mere bystanders.

The physicians have prescribed medications for them, which they have to take regularly. Despite taking these regularly, there is no improvement. Quite the contrary, their condition worsens.

Because of all these symptoms, the family also begins to be very concerned about them. Family and friends pity the patient. They sincerely do their best to take care of them now that they are ill, possibly even seriously ill and suffering, having to renounce everything that they were fond of. The compassion and care of family and friends even goes so far that they advise them to stay away from any kind of activity. Helpful and ready to make sacrifices, family members and friends stand by them. Despite their helpfulness and good wishes, resignation and despair slowly and steadily creep up on them. Because of the seemingly prolonged illness, family and friends become used to the fact that these once cheerful and healthy people are now ill, perhaps even incurably ill. As time goes by, even their helpfulness diminishes and the patients, the invalids, feel left alone. It has now become a matter of course to the family that they are ill and need to take things easy, that they need kindness, leniency and help.

The friends who at first visited them daily, now come less and less. They hardly allow them to participate in their lives. Now and then, as it so happens, they take their sick friends along to their weekly sports and games. Now they can only be spectators and observers. The sick ones now realize that life is showing them other pathways. The seemingly sick people, who, with their senses, were and still are closely attached to the world and its pleasures, feel disadvantaged by fate. They fall more and more into resignation and their minds become duller and duller. They complain that from one day to the next they have had to give up everything that made their lives worth living and rich in content. Disappointment with their fellow people who no longer pay enough attention to them leads to further resignation, despair and apathy.

The result of this deep resignation, which is based on a wrong attitude toward life and way of dealing with it, is thoughts of envy. They envy every person's health, happiness and joys.

From these feelings and thoughts of envy, soon develops hatred toward their family and friends, who, they believe, have left them to their fate. Jealousy, inner distress, despondency and inner turmoil wear down their nervous system, thus worsening the condition of their illness that was initially merely an indisposition.

What happened here?

These world-oriented persons had paid scant attention to the laws of God and hardly given them any significance. They relied totally on the physicians' diagnosis and opinion. The consequence of this was that their life changed from one day to the next. According to the medical advice, the hitherto healthy people had to immediately change their diet, give up sports and games and take medications according to exact instructions. The engine running at high performance—the human body, over-strained by competitive sports and very rich food, by alcohol and tobacco—was immobilized from one day to the next, following the medical diagnosis. The so-called illness should have been brought to a standstill and cured in this way. The physicians relied solely on their diagnosis; they did not, however, take into consideration the situation of the persons in question, especially their world of thoughts, their former lifestyle, and its resulting prestige-oriented attitude. Through the abrupt interruption of all habits, their organism suffered an enormous shock. The high-performance machine, the person, was brought to a full stop from one hour to the next.

A comparison:

A high-performance machine, regardless for what purpose it was built by human hands, may never be abruptly brought down to half its performance. It is gradually switched down to a lower performance.

The same procedure should be used on the physical body, which can be compared to a high-performance machine.

The body of a human being is an energy body, because everything is energy. Through the shock of learning that they might be ill, even suffering, and that they have to give up from one day to the next everything that made life worth living, these people lost their balance. The engines, the human beings, were abruptly throttled back to half-performance. Through the shock of now having to give up everything, they reached the sphere of thoughts of envy and hatred, a phase in which they came to consider self-destruction. As a result, the vibration of their body lowered more and more. Through this wrong way of thinking, they were seized by thought complexes that intensified their negative thinking even more.

For your better understanding, let it be repeated:

Everything is based on vibration. Like always attracts like.

The patients' hate-filled and self-destructive way of thinking tensed their nervous system more and more, and thus, the fine nerves in the organs as well, particularly those already weakened. The negative thoughts had a disturbing effect on their blood circulation and on their heart.

Since the body rhythm sank very quickly and the whole body slipped into lower zones of vibration, neither the various natural remedies nor pharmaceutical medications could provide any significant relief, or even healing. The difference between the patients' vibration and the vibration of the remedies was too great. Both the pharmaceutical medications and natural remedies had a more destructive effect on the body than a beneficial and healing one. The negative effects of the medications became stronger, affecting other weak and susceptible organs, as well. The patients' condition worsened.

Because of the mistaken actions of both physicians and patients, the initial indisposition became an illness with corresponding consequences. The negative feelings and thoughts of those seeking help, the fear and worry for their life, contributed decisively to turning the initial indisposition into an illness. Because of a wrong way of thinking, speaking and acting, the nervous system became ever more tense, and thus, also the tiniest nerves that permeate the organs.

Highly tensed nerves secrete toxins that, depending on the vibration of the body of an individual, either detrimentally affect susceptible organs or poison the whole body.

I, the Inner Physician and Healer, Christ, your Redeemer, call these toxins "neurotoxins." They can influence and impair a person's organism to such a degree that it will hardly react to natural remedies or pharmaceutical medications.

Through the secretion of neurotoxins, a so-called nerve fever can develop, which, via the central nervous system, sets all the nerves in vibration, so that the entire organism is heated up, that is, becomes overheated. It is this congestion and warmth, or even heat, that harms the fine tissues in the body. This unusual and unhealthy body heat shows that the nervous system is

suffering greatly from the pressure of both consciousness and subconscious.

Outer symptoms are bouts of perspiration that occur at the slightest agitation. The person in question thus excretes many trace elements, so that finally their body becomes weaker and weaker and susceptible to other illnesses. These signs may also be an indication for one of the most serious illnesses to hit people in manifold ways and forms.

What I gave and am still giving in revelation here provides insight into the manifold occurrences and situations that take place at every moment in the material world. The previous example showed that the result of a perhaps quite small soul burden that was released during the night and appeared in the body as an indisposition upon awakening—through wrong thinking, through a thoughtless and wrong diagnosis and advice—can develop into an illness that may lead to lingering illness or even physical death.

Whatever remained in the soul through wrong behavior or was even reinforced there is taken by the soul into the soul realms after its disembodiment, after its physical death. With the same features and characteristics, it can enter this world again at another time or epoch and in another body.

O human being, recognize yourself and be on your guard! Never allow an indisposition to become an illness, because you look at the indisposition in fear, thus affirming it as an illness.

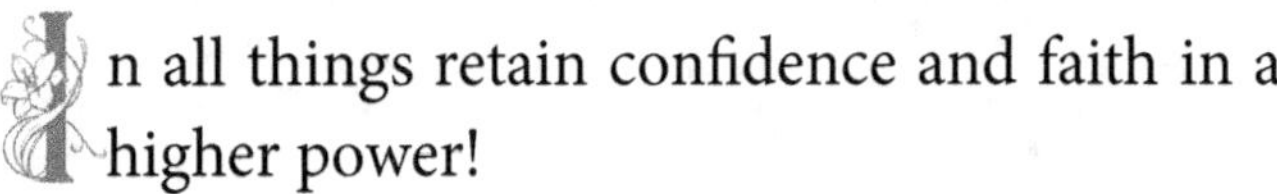

In all things retain confidence and faith in a higher power!

Maintain a healthy optimism despite temporary physical suffering and difficulties. Affirm the positive in you! Affirm the health and strength of your soul and of your body. Through this, you address the positive in the negative, which, in time, will outweigh and transform the still active negativity into the positive. If you promote the positive aspects that are present as a force in everything negative, then the positive becomes effective and cancels out the negative, the contrary.

There are two possibilities open to people: They can attribute an illness to themselves, thus promoting it, or they can stimulate healing and become healthy. Both forces are in the soul or human being as predispositions. These possibilities are chances for each person in each incarnation—until the soul has become a spirit being again, once more living in its primordial homeland, where absolute peace and harmony are the basic principles of love.

The law of cause and effect is effective in both soul and person. What people think and how they live is carried out in the effect.

Those who have not and do not practice self-control and self-examination in their life also do not know themselves. Those who don't know themselves don't know their neighbor either. Therefore, they are incapable of changing their life.

Those who strive for a positive life, who affirm the good and refine their senses also know their body and can direct it accordingly.

Imitators accept everything that is said and recommended to them. For them, everything their neighbor says or that is recommended for their body is reality.

If physicians or psychologists never recognize themselves, they will not recognize a patient and person seeking help either. They look only at the external appearance, failing to understand the cause, what actually lies before them. They will continue to seek in the dark until they have examined themselves and it has become brighter and clearer in them.

To lead a conscious life, in order to be able to truly help one's neighbor, those wanting to help first have to examine themselves and change their life toward the spiritual. Only then is it possible to recognize their neighbors and to help them in the right way.

The transformation from ignorance to self-recognition and self-experience does not happen from one moment to the next, but step by step—depending on the measure to which the individuals themselves practice self-control and self-examination and actualization. This leads to a complete change, all the way to the purely spiritual.

Those who recognize themselves change themselves; their life will gradually become positive and conscious.

Just as people think, they are. And just as they think and live, they react.

With their thoughts that are their life, they influence their entire organism, each organ and each cell of their body.

If someone has hitherto paid no attention to their thoughts and to their way of life, and if today, they begin to think positively, they cannot expect that their organism—the cells, organs, muscles, glands and hormones—will adjust from one day to the next and immediately react positively. The adjustment has to be gradual. For people turned to without, it is not possible from one day to the next to fashion their way of feeling, thinking and living to be only positive and selfless.

All growth is subject to fluctuation. This will also be experienced by the person who turns away from all-too-human thinking to think and live lawfully, that is, spiritually.

Therefore, it would be just as wrong to put the organism on a diet from one day to the next. The cell tissues would give up, since they are accustomed to another rhythm of life and another kind of nourishment. This inappropriate action would have a negative effect on the person—for instance, in the form of fatigue, exhaustion, listlessness, depression and, not lastly, of aggression. In many cases, these consequences would also be directed against their fellow people who may have burdened the patients with advice to change their diet from one day to the next.

The discontent of those concerned not only has an effect on their family, but also on friends and acquaintances. People who have everything taken from them from one day to the next become resentful and turn into tyrants. It is the cell tissues, the consciousness and subconscious of the cells, which rebel in the human being, demanding what they have long since grown accustomed to. This is why the organism should be adjusted slowly and without fanaticism.

All difficulties, problems and illnesses are based on something that lies in the soul. Every illness has a cause that lies in the soul.

The physician and the patient should make a joint effort to find the cause of an illness, which always lies in the spiritual spheres. The source of all indispositions, illnesses, worries and blows of fate lies, as stated, in the spiritual realm.

Therefore, those seeking healing are advised, among other things, to pay more attention to the reactions of their body. The body, the organism, calls for what it wants or needs via the sensory organs. With the right kind of training for life that leads to health, the demands and desires of the cell tissues and of the body are only partially fulfilled. This means that whatever the cell tissue wants, but is not lawful, is gradually reduced. This is a slow adjustment from old human customs and habits to a lawful life.

The cells and organs give a signal via the sensory organs. They inform the alert person what they are lacking.

Thus, via the senses, the organism reveals, for instance, what nutritive substances it needs to create the conditions necessary for healing from within. This is why this method of healing should be called: "Healing by the Spirit, God."

The body prepares itself for healing by the Spirit if the person pays attention to the signals of the organism.

If spirit, soul and body are largely in consonance, then healing by the Spirit, God, can take place.

If people reduce the intake of such luxury items as alcohol and tobacco—which often poison the body by tensing the nerves so that they secrete neurotoxins—and if they try to think positively, that is, divinely, they will not ignore the signals of their body. They will then give their organism what it needs to prepare itself for healing by the Spirit.

The physicians, whom I also call "apostles of health," first endeavor to detoxify the body of the person seeking healing before prescribing the appropriate natural remedies—for a tense nervous system and an over-acidified body poisoned by neurotoxins, can hardly absorb the natural remedies or make use of them. In these cases, they leave the organism without any positive effect.

Therefore, the physicians should slowly readjust the organism by deacidifying and detoxifying it. They endeavor to treat and stimulate the cell tissues in such a way that they give corresponding signals to the patients, so that they may experience for themselves what is good or not so good for them.

Only once the body shows a reaction are the cell tissues and organs ready to cooperate on their own during the healing. Only then, can the organism appreciate the correct and healthy nourishment, knowing how to make use of it in such a way that the sick organs are able to absorb the appropriate substances from it. The same applies to natural remedies. An active organism makes good use of both food and remedies.

There is an extensive therapy for preparing the body for spiritual healing which I, the Spirit of Christ, explain in this revelation only in general terms. Every living organism manifests itself in the way in which it is programmed. If the program that has been entered into it is wrong, then it must slowly and carefully be reprogrammed positively. This means that the person must affirm and lead a positive life.

This seemingly new and profound method of healing for the people of the New Era comes from the eternal truth—which was merely buried under the intellect and vain delusion.

Harmony brings about health.
More about neurotoxins

Recognize that the nerves are important components of the human body. If more attention is paid to the nerves from the very beginning of treatment, the organism receives the first impulse for positive participation. The patients relax and are willing to positively change their previous milieu that has shaped them, and to draw the corresponding consequences.

The nervous system is mainly burdened by wrong thinking, but also by wrong nutrition. Large quantities of food also burden the nervous system. It becomes tense and eventually secretes toxins that poison the whole organism, if they are not recognized in time and the body is not detoxified and deacidified.

Neurotoxins can also cause paralysis. If the nerves remain tense for a prolonged period of time and if the person leads an unhealthy life, consuming a lot of meat, fish, nicotine, alcohol and the like, then various forms of paralysis of differing intensity can arise.

Calcification, deposits in the blood vessels, can also be produced by a constant tension of the nerves, which, in addition, also secrete neurotoxins.

Neurotoxins can also have a contrary effect on medications and natural remedies that have been taken: They change the characteristics of the plant and pharmaceutical substances and can thus lead to side-effects.

People also talk about so-called "soul-toxins," although in so doing, they equate the soul with the nervous system. The soul, the burdened spirit body that dwells in the human being, does not secrete toxins. However, the causes created by a person are stored in the soul and come into effect in the body.

To become and remain healthy, people should strive for harmony on and in themselves and in their immediate surroundings. Harmony brings about health.

Human beings should also economize their energies. For example, wrongful thinking, speaking, acting and too much talking—above all, unessential speaking—cost the organism more energy than several hours of concentrated heavy labor.

Those who make the worries and problems of their neighbor their own by pondering over the behavior of others, by talking to them about it for hours, perhaps even getting annoyed because old difficulties and problems are re-freshed again and again, open their own door to these problem vibrations of their neighbors and make them their own. They open themselves through their annoyance with their neighbor because the latter keeps talking about the same worries and problems.

The reasons why people keep talking about their worries and problems can be manifold. One person, for instance, wants to increase their sense of self-importance, the other wants to be pitied.

It is not lawful for someone to keep listening to the same problem over and over again and to keep discussing it with the problem-laden person. Energy is drawn from the listener and repetitions debilitate the latter's nervous system. In a weakened listener, this can cause an indis-position or even an illness.

Such circumstances could lead to the fact that the those who wanted to help and keep listening to the same problems over and over again, reach the point where their nervous system tenses up and secretes toxins, which then attack their organism and could trigger an illness.

Everyone is called upon to help and to serve their neighbor as far as they are able to and based on their spiritual growth and external possibilities.

However, there is no spiritual commandment that a person has to listen to the difficulties and problems of their fellow people over and over again. Those who keep talking about the same worries and problems do not want to tackle them and overcome them at all, but rather want to show off with them, to aggrandize themselves or elicit pity.

Those who serve selflessly are protected from every refutation. Nevertheless, they are also called upon to economize their soul energies and their physical energies.

However, someone whose motive for serving is ambition, praise and recognition, thereby misusing their spiritual and physical energies, will suffer from it.

Those who listen to the worries and problems of their neighbor again and again, getting annoyed and upset over it, without telling the person concerned to let go of the past and unlawful aspects or to clear them up, infect themselves with the vibrations of the problem-laden person.

Furthermore, the law says: Help your neighbors in word and deed to the best of your knowledge and conscience, yet do not impose your help on them or force them to accept what you think is right for them.

If your neighbors are not willing to follow your good advice and accept your help, if they just want to increase their sense of self-importance, then let them be but do not repudiate them. If you have explained their situation to them according to the laws of life and they refuse to accept a lawful explanation and help, then be silent and pray all the more for them.

Every person who lives in the endeavor to actualize the eternal laws is called upon to clarify the law of cause and effect to their neighbors, and that they should take everything that is all-too-human, that troubles them—worry, suffering, problems, indispositions and illnesses—and surrender them to the eternal Spirit, the Inner Physician and Healer, and leave them there.

The knowing person should also explain to those seeking help about forgiveness and asking for forgiveness, so that in this way, their neighbors may also be led to self-recognition.

The All-Highest has given free will to every soul and to every human being as their heritage. Therefore, do not force your neighbor to do your will. Every human being should recognize that their very own way of thinking and acting is the motive force in their life.

Recognize that a person's today is their tomorrow.

This means that whatever they carry out today that is good, less good, or even unlawful, shapes their future: their continuing life on Earth or even their life as a soul in the spheres of purification.

Each minute is precious for the human being. Therefore, O human being, make use of every moment, of every minute!

The soul is in the earthly garment to learn to live in a lawful way. Those who do not live lawfully, that is, who do not ennoble their thinking, their wanting and striving, do not learn to think, speak and act in a divine way either, and their life is one of mere vegetating. They waste the time and energies of this existence.

Every person is the forger of their own fate. The anvil is the correspondences in soul and person: the feelings, the inclinations, the desires and wanting.

On top of the anvil, on top of the correspondences, further inclinations, drives, feelings, thoughts, words and actions may be added, according to the person's way of thinking, speaking and acting. Therefore, every person forges their own fate and shapes their own life.

Those who live with the world are also subject to the capriciousness of the world. They are the plaything of their own thoughts and desires, and even of the thoughts and desires of their fellow people.

People will have to wade through the morass created by themselves until they attain recognition and actualization, thereby awakening to higher spirituality.

The difference between Redeemer and Comforter

Those who live in Me, the omnipotence, will receive comfort, salvation and redemption, for I Am not only the Redeemer of all souls and human beings, but also the Comforter in suffering, pain and need. Comforter and Redeemer are two forces in the one power, in Me, the Christ-Power.

The part-power of the primordial power is the power of redemption. From it, flows the comforting power, which gives comfort and help to the suffering soul and enslaved human being.

The redeeming power frees the willing person who has turned to Me of the ties to opinions, concepts, philosophies and forms. It raises the awakened soul longing for God to the primordial power and gradually leads it back to the bosom of God.

The comforting power receives the soul that is still weak and bound and the human being who, despite spiritual admonition and instruction, has not yet awakened and feels no longing for God. These are souls and human beings who, as a consequence of their burdens, are still too weak to recognize and understand the truth so that they can take the first step toward Me.

The comforting power gives consolation and help to the weakened soul, to the sick and suffering human being burdened by fate. It gives strength to bear one's fate. In both soul and person, it brings about a relief and brightening of the state of mind. Over and over again, it lets the enslaved soul and suffering person draw new hope.

The glorious divine love of the Father works in manifold ways through Me, His Son, who, as Jesus of Nazareth, was the personification of God's Mercy.

The comforting power also is active in all souls and people who have to suffer from the effect of a heavy soul debt that cannot be transformed yet, because it serves the soul for spiritual development and maturity.

The power of the Comforter is also granted to those souls which, in this or in a further life on Earth, return to the same level of consciousness again and again, so as to expiate a heavy burden. They are the souls in the earthly garment that, during several incarnations, are expiating one and the same soul debt that they inflicted on themselves during one of their prior existences.

Depending on its intensity, a heavy soul debt may not be paid off in one lifetime on Earth, because the physical energies would not be sufficient. In other words, the human being could not bear the burden all at once.

If the comforting and healing power contained in the Redeemer-power were not a help to the still weak souls and people, many would be broken by their fate.

God is love. All human beings and souls receive this love—according to their spiritual development and maturity.

The part-stream from the Redeemer-power —the power of comfort and healing—does not yet directly stimulate evolution in soul and person. Instead, it supports, comforts, helps and heals, so that the weak soul and suffering person may receive strength to then be able to walk the path of evolution.

Once the shackles of the great soul burden have been loosened and the spiritual life begins to germinate in soul and person, the redeeming and uplifting power then starts working more intensely to lead soul and person to higher spirituality.

A great burden of the soul may also have accumulated over several lives on Earth, during which a person committed the same mistakes over and over again. It may possibly have to be paid off in parts over several incarnations. Souls and human beings who are still under these effects will make no great progress on the path of evolution during this time.

Burdens of the soul and person can be transformed and dissolved by Me, the Spirit of Christ, only when soul and person are willing to repent and to forgive through self-experience and self-recognition, and to grow and mature spiritually by actualizing the holy laws.

Only when the old, often repeated, same and like faults, weaknesses and sins are no longer committed, will soul and person walk the path of spiritual evolution.

Since many people are stubborn and obstinate, they have a hard time bearing their self-imposed burdens.

The Comforter, the Holy Spirit, is also the Redeemer, the Spirit of Christ, who works in manifold ways and means to support the souls and people, to help them and lead them home.

I Am in God, My Father, this power that comforts, helps, heals and redeems.

I Am.

Advice from the divine Love and Wisdom for people of the Spirit

The Spirit is in everything that is, that lives. The eternal Spirit, the absolute life, is also the Comforter, Healer and Redeemer of every soul and of every person.

The divine life is indirectly at work in the person who is still tied to the wheel of reincarnation by those soul burdens that have not yet been expiated.

The eternal Spirit is harmony.

Harmony expresses itself in colors, shapes, sounds, fragrances, movements and in words. The more soul and person live in harmony with God, the finer is the radiation of both soul and body. The life of such people then expresses itself in their even disposition, in the harmonious colors and forms of their clothing, in the delicate, discrete nuances of fragrances they choose, in their graceful, aesthetic movements, and in their spiritual, selfless and caring language. This person is then in harmony.

The field of vibration of both soul and person is comprised of the feelings, thoughts, words and deeds that the soul has imposed on itself, that is, has acquired over the course of its incarnations, its journeys on Earth.

Until all shadows have been eliminated in soul and person, the wayfarer on the path toward the Absolute experiences highs and lows, joy and suffering, spiritual darkness and enlightenment.

The interactions in the life of a human being, the large fluctuations between joy and suffering, between depression and hope, indicate that the person is still under the influence of the stars and under the influence of the surroundings. The more these fluctuations, these highs and lows, diminish in intensity and frequency, the freer and more light-filled soul and person become.

People have to ennoble their thoughts, stirrings and inclinations and refine their senses in order to grow and mature spiritually. Without self-control, without monitoring themselves, both soul and person merely vegetate. They let costly time go by, by living blindly in the shadow of their ego without heeding the eternal laws.

Free will from God means: I, your Redeemer, servant and helper, can stand by you and take your evil from you only when you turn to Me. Mere lip-prayers are not enough, but only the heartfelt prayer and a change in your way of thinking, living and acting from what is human to the spiritual. Without your own effort, there is no actualization and fulfillment of the holy laws, and no path to the kingdom of the inner being.

Let it be repeated for better understanding: What gains entrance in people, what annoys them, that corresponds to their nature; that is what they themselves are.

However, those who want to spiritualize their life, to find their way out of the vibrational field of unlawful influences—out of the magnetic field of human thinking, feeling, and wanting—in order to gain strength, healing and redemption in both soul and body, should pay attention to the following:

Every pointless, brooding, aimless thought and every useless word is wasted energy.

Those who do not have their life, their thoughts and actions under control expand and strengthen their negative field of vibration and perhaps reach even lower spheres of vibration, depending on the pathways of thought their life follows. There they increase the burdens of their soul until this field of vibration becomes effective and then breaks in over them as an illness or blow of fate.

Once the soul starts to break loose from the wheel of reincarnation, and once a person has largely paid off all the burdens of their soul through a life oriented to God and the eternal laws and by virtue of My grace, this person is then free, harmonious and spiritually balanced. Such people are positive toward their neighbor and toward all things and occurrences. They know they are secure in the bosom of the Godhead.

People of the Spirit know the law of cause and effect: In many cases, because of their wrong thinking and acting, they had to go through much suffering and thus came to realize that what people sow, they will reap.

By reason of the lessons learned through personal experience, by way of sowing and reaping, they have grown wise. They are no longer imitators. They may well weigh what is false and what is true. They may well listen to the arguments, objections and advice of their fellow people and know how to classify them accordingly, but they are not affected by them. They do not become upset and do not reply with opposing arguments and cynical statements, but give an answer that is from the eternal law.

People of the Spirit will respond to all-too-human remarks, to cynicism and the like only when there is a need to clarify the situation—but they do not defend themselves. They do, however, raise pertinent objections that are meant to give their neighbors food for thought without hurting them.

People of the Spirit have a highly developed ability to empathize, because they no longer think of themselves, because they are free of base thoughts and desires. Their freedom and unity with the divine enable them to see things and occurrences as they are and not as they seem to be. What seems to be can deceive—but not what is.

They draw from their opened spirit consciousness and, for this reason, will stand by their neighbor in word and deed, insofar as the neighbor can understand and accept it in the right way. They find the right measure for everyone. They speak only what is necessary and lawful. They do not go beyond their neighbor's capacity of comprehension.

Spiritual people will follow the well-intentioned advice of their fellow person only if this advice is in accordance with the law. They will not set their fellow person straight. They thank their neighbor for the well-intentioned advice but do not think about it any longer if, by virtue of their own spiritual development, they have come to realize that the advice is not in accordance with the eternal law.

They should also refrain from talking with others about the advice they received from a fellow person. What their neighbor has confided or communicated to them concerns only God and His child, and not a third or fourth party—unless it is necessary to help clear up a certain matter.

About fear and forgiveness

These smaller and larger remarks, instructions and indications given by Me, the Spirit of Christ, are spiritual principles from the divine Love and Wisdom. The one who heeds them and live accordingly finds the key to the door of life, which I Am.

A person whose thinking and acting is in accordance with the law becomes a bearer of the energy of divine life.

As long as people keep thinking about trivial things, talking at great length or even getting annoyed about them, they are merely moving their own correspondences, their ego, in their inner being. These are indicators of God's indirect guidance.

People who are preoccupied with themselves, who talk a lot about themselves and think about their own concerns are still under the causal law. They are indirectly guided by the eternal law via the radiation of the stars. Whatever it is that upsets people shows that the same or like things are still in them.

What is base has no power of its own unless people lend it energy through their wrong way of thinking and acting, because thoughts, words and actions are energies.

Many people are afraid of illness and blows of fate. Like every thought, every word and action, fear is a magnetic force. People attract what they are afraid of and what they move in thoughts and words.

Fear and every thought, every word and every action have a cause.

A cause of fear, for instance, can be the concealment of things and occurrences: The neighbor is not supposed to know what is going on in the fearful person. Those who are afraid want to keep or hide something.

Fear may also be based on past failures, blows of fate, worries, suffering, disappointments and disputes that the fearful ones have not yet overcome, or for which they have not yet forgiven their neighbor. Fearful people are afraid that the same or like things could happen to them again.

Fear can also emanate from the soul garments in which there is still something unatoned for. A fearful person should not brush this aside by saying that it might come from former lives, because the life of an individual is a whole. There is no separation between here and there, between the still burdened past and the present. The past touches the present, provided there is still something that has not been atoned for.

Fear as such can also be a sign that the past, the unatoned, is emerging and should now be cleared up.

Fear is no more than a thought complex through which envy, greed, hatred and jealousy may be expressed. Such thoughts, words and deeds, which have not yet been atoned for and may have occurred in past lives, now touch soul and person in this existence. They want to draw the person's attention to what is waiting to be cleared up.

Fearfulness, expressions of conscience or unlawful thoughts can often be admonitions. They stimulate people to forgive what they have recognized. Those who recognize and accept these admonishers, who clear up what has been recognized, walk on the path to God and will no longer have to endure or suffer many things.

The request for forgiveness of one's neighbor or of a soul should take place via Me, the

Christ, the Redeemer of all people and souls. In this way, those asking for forgiveness are also protected: They cannot be touched by souls that may have been asked for forgiveness, because the person asking for forgiveness is under spiritual protection.

The guardian spirit can also touch a human being and appear as admonisher when the person thinks and speaks wrongly or gives instructions and does things that are not according to the law. Someone who is alert will react immediately.

People do not always know for what they should ask forgiveness or what they should forgive. There are impulses that penetrate their world of feelings, touching them so that suddenly they feel: "I ought to ask for forgiveness or forgive; but I don't know whom or why I should ask for forgiveness, let alone forgive." An alert person will carry this out through Me, the Christ, thus finding inner freedom and peace.

Those who know about these lawful principles will recognize the signs that become evident in their world of feelings. It does not matter whether or not they know the person they may have wronged or who has wronged them. They do not ask whether they were souls or human beings who lived with them in this or former lives, and who have been hurt, mistreated or insulted by them, or who insulted or mistreated them. Those who feel that they ought to ask for forgiveness or to forgive should make no distinction as to whether they know the person concerned or not. Through Me, the Christ, they should let their inner request for forgiveness flow into the universe or forgive through Me.

I am the way, the truth and the life. Those who ask for forgiveness or forgive through Me, the Christ, can be confident that it will come at the right hour and time and release everything that has been bound.

With all your heart, ask your neighbor for forgiveness and you, forgive, too! A wrong done or a cause is never one-sided. If your neighbor has wronged you, forgive and do not ask if the neighbor who is just as involved in the cause has already forgiven you. In so doing, the soul purifies itself and can receive more light and spirituality. Through this, both soul and person become kind, loving and understanding.

Thus, whatever acts on the human being from without or from within and causes restlessness and aggression in the person is a trait of the human ego, for like always moves like.

The time of grace

God's love flows into this world in manifold ways, as does the heightened time of grace for His children. It is called a time of grace.

The time of grace is granted to a person who wants to strive for a life that is pleasing to God, who endeavors, over and over again, to put the eternal laws into practice. The heightened time of grace supports the first smaller and larger steps of the soul and person on the way to perfection.

However, the period of grace is limited to a certain time. It works and offers protection to the person until the first firm steps on the way to God, the life, have been accomplished through recognition and actualization. If through actualization, the protected person is largely oriented to the goal of thinking and living divinely, then the time of grace, the heightened grace period, gradually recedes. The wayfarers on the path to the goal, to God, continue to receive strength from the All-power so that by continuing to recognize themselves, they can repent and discard their faults. Yet the protective shell of the time of grace no longer surrounds them.

During the time of grace, both the inner power, the Holy Spirit, and the guardian spirit try, via inner impulses and via guidance by way of second and third persons, to admonish the person in the time of grace to adopt a correct spiritual behavior.

The Spirit of God and the guardian spirit become more active via the conscience. The conscience is a function of certain brain cells and of the nervous system.

However, if the person complies with the awakening impulse from the divine for only a short time, if the lawful teachings and guidance are accepted only temporarily—perhaps merely listened to—and if the person then returns to the world with all its habits and vices, then the increased protection withdraws.

People reject God's help through their behavior. This does not mean that God also withdraws His hand from His child. God continues to guide His child. But the help for the spiritual start, the strengthened protection, withdraws. The Spirit respects the free will of His children.

The beneficial effect of water

Everything is energy.

Just as your thoughts have an effect in and on you, building up and harmonizing your nervous system, the sounding board of your body, or creating tensions and dissonances in it—so can water do the same on and in you: It harmonizes you or it causes disharmonies in and on you.

Just as your thoughts flow into you or out of you, a stream of water that is directed over your nervous system can also have an effect.

Water is the driving element. It causes you to reach a higher vibration; it harmonizes your nervous system, thus stimulating you to a positive way of thinking. But you have to contribute to this: You have to let go of what preoccupies you and surrender it to Me or, depending on the burden, clear it up and put it in order.

A warm stream of water, not too hot, that is adjusted to your body temperature, can get rid of many things externally and stabilize and recharge your magnetic field, the aura, in a positive sense.

Thus, if the stream of water is properly directed and applied, the water magnetizes and energizes the body. It relaxes the nervous system that contains the life force in and around it.

Depending on the tension and restlessness of your body, let a warm stream of water flow over your back for several minutes or even a little longer. Point the nice warm stream of water to your hairline at the back of your neck. Relax while doing this and release from your consciousness all base feelings and thoughts, everything that the day brought that disturbed you. Instead of troubled thoughts replace them with highly vibrating thoughts of peace, joy, of unity with Me, your Lord and God.

If you cannot attain harmony, then listen to harmonious music that puts you in a good mood while the water flows, starting from your neck over your nervous system.

With this treatment both the circulation and the spirit power in the body, in the nerves and in the cells are stimulated.

Recognize that the blood circulation functions well only when the nervous system is relaxed, and the forces of the Spirit can flow increasingly.

Very cold gushes of water are not in accordance with the law. They do not relax or harmonize, but cause tension in the organism and lead to tension and disturbances in the nervous and connective tissues, which, sooner or later, may cause nervous disorders or bring about other causes and effects. As already revealed, a person should not drink ice-cold beverages either, because these are not good for the organism.

Nor should a person go into cold water with a heated body. Many people know that this shock can lead to cardiac arrest. The same is true with a jet or gush of water that is too cold.

Therefore, do not shock your body. Every cold shock causes tension in the nervous system. Water can be relaxing and beneficial for the organism if properly applied.

If water is applied as a therapy, it can have not only a beneficial effect on the organism but can also ease tensions in the soul so that the spirit power can flow more strongly, providing relief and healing. However, everything must be done in the right measure.

Just as very cold water leads to tension, water that is too hot can also strain the nervous system and eventually cause the vessels to slacken.

After water therapy go into inner stillness and let the energies working in you develop to their full capacity. If possible, lie flat on your bed; cover your body with light, warm blankets and remain in this position, relaxed and aware of the inner power, aware that I, the Spirit, the Inner Physician and Healer, am active in you. When you rise from your resting place after a few minutes, give thanks to God, honor and praise His name. Through this, you will have a positive influence on your cells, on your organs and blood circulation. In other words, you stimulate your body, causing the life force in you to increase.

Water therapy, properly applied, is a means of help and healing. Recognize that it brings you strengthening and healing. It is important, however, that your thoughts and feelings are with God, your Lord, who is also active working in the water.

An even more effective method of help and healing through the application of water is by addressing the consciousness centers with a weaker stream of water.

However, this therapy should be carried out only by knowing, wise people who know the law of life. Someone who conducts this targeted water treatment inadequately can possibly do more harm than good.

The water therapy should also be accompanied with positive powers of thought.

Water therapy alone does not bring lasting relief and healing. Both must take place: water therapy and a change of thoughts and actions. The people must affirm the forces of life that flow in their inner being and are also active in the water.

Everything is energy. Every stream of power can be strengthened or weakened through the power of thought.

Similarly, a stream of water, which is also energy, can be charged with increased power or reduced in its effectiveness if the thoughts of the person seeking healing are not in order. Here again, the attitude of the person is decisive.

Life, all Being, serves humankind. Sun, moon and stars, all the heavenly bodies of the material and the part-material universe bring about help and guidance in souls, human beings and part-material beings. They also move the predispositions in incarnated souls, in human beings, motivating soul and person—even through illness and blows of fate—to come to recognize and actualize the laws of God. Thus, human beings are the architect of their fate and the builder of their life.

People who use and apply the energies in a positive sense for the benefit of humankind will also benefit themselves. Therefore, those who use water in the correct way, increasing the energy of water through the power of thought, stimulate the atoms of their own body. Through the water therapy, they bring them into a higher vibration, which may, in turn, bring about inner and outer healing.

If the energy potential of the soul and body is highly vibrating, that is, if the person is positively oriented, then the energy potential of the water will also adapt to the body much faster. Then even after a short application, there is an increased interaction, a communication of the forces of water and body, which stimulates the atomic structure of the body. If people have a negative or pessimistic attitude toward life, the water may still vitalize and refresh them and stimulate their organism; but this effect will not be lasting and will bring little success, because the deep effect is missing.

All powers of infinity want to serve humankind. The eternal powers are the law, God.

The spiritual law says: Like draws to like; they mutually reinforce one another and bring about what human beings mentally orient themselves to.

The quanta, the spiritual part-powers,
are the spiritual bearers of energy:
They transfer the spirit power into matter,
into the material atoms

People's attitude toward life and their way of life are decisive for the soul. The soul is magnetized according to the thinking and living of the person. Therefore, what people think and speak and how they act is registered by the soul.

Both soul and person consist of atoms. The soul consists of spiritual atoms, the human being of material atoms. And yet, spiritual energy radiates into the material, into the power that has been transformed down. This happens via so-called quanta.

356

Quanta are spiritual part-powers. They are the building blocks for the material life. Via these spiritual part-powers, the quanta, the spirit power flows into the physical body. Prior to this, however, the sub-quanta, as I call them, come into effect. They bring about the influx of the spirit power into the quanta. They cannot be perceived by human beings because they are the pure spiritual substance of the material atoms.

The material atom is dependent on the spirit power that consists of spiritual atoms. The sub-quanta are spiritual atoms that extend into matter. The spiritual part-powers, the quanta, are partly pure spirit power, then again transformed down energy, that is, matter—it depends on the person's attitude toward life and lifestyle. This also applies to the quanta in all material forms. Thus, how people think and act, so do they affect their environment.

The spirit power flows into the organism of a person as follows:

The spiritual part-powers, the quanta, are dependent on the absolute spirit power, the seven basic powers of creation, which are called the natures and attributes of God. Without the spiritual power nothing can exist.

I deliberately repeat, over and over again, that everything is energy: Every thought, every word and every action is energy. Since no energy is lost, it must be noticeable either in, on or around the body or in the atmosphere.

Thus, people's way of thinking, speaking and acting determines the number and effectiveness of the quanta. Hence, people themselves determine the intensity and number of spiritual part-powers, of quanta. For this reason, in the material atoms of the human organism either a low or a higher number of spiritual part-powers may be present and effective.

As already revealed, people's way of thinking, speaking and acting is decisive. If they are very materially oriented, that is, if their attitude toward life and their way of life are focused solely on matter, if their thoughts are negative, envious and malicious, if they are contentious, jealous and in conflict with their neighbor, all these human aspects have an effect on the formation and activity of the quanta.

A materially oriented way of life results in a very low level of activity of the spiritual part-powers, the quanta. There are fewer spiritual part-powers effective, and the active quanta are predominantly visible, that is, material.

The more people are spiritualized, in other words, the more they have turned toward the divine law by putting it into practice, the more spiritual part-powers are in them, in their atomic structure, and are effective mainly in the sphere of invisibility. The result is the following:

The more spiritual part-powers, quanta, are present in the atoms of a person, the healthier, more flexible and spiritually active the person is.

For the better understanding of my children on Earth, I repeat: The spiritual part-powers, the quanta, originate from the five spiritual types of atoms. As revealed, they are, among other things, the bearers of life for the material atoms.

The spiritual atoms, the spiritual atomic energy that is set in the particles of the soul, are in continual activity.

The Primordial Central Sun radiates into infinity via the secondary primordial suns, also called prism suns, which disperse the primordial light into seven times seven spectral colors. In this way, the Primordial Central Sun reaches every form of life, including soul and person, via the prism suns.

The spirit beings, souls and human beings belong respectively to one of the seven prism suns, which are also called the natures and attributes of God. Depending on the mentality of the spirit being and of the soul, they are allocated to a nature or attribute, a prism sun.

As revealed, every spirit being and every soul has in itself the incorruptible core of being, which is also called the spiritual heart of the spiritual body. The core of being is oriented to one of the seven prism suns and, via this, to the Primordial Central Sun. Every soul and every spirit being is linked to that prism sun to which the nature and attribute of the spirit being or soul belong. No soul can change its divine nature or attribute, which is effective in it in a formative way. It is the soul's spiritual birth-ray.

The more the spiritual atomic energy in the particles of the spiritual body—also called soul—is oriented toward the core of being, the more active it is. According to its increased activity, it attracts more energy from infinity. This then has a positive effect in both soul and body.

These increased spiritual-energetic forces are not only active in the soul. A part of these spiritual energies flows via the quanta into the material atoms, into the cells, organs, glands, hormones, and muscles—into the entire organism of the person. Everything happens according to the heavenly order. As people think and live, they receive accordingly.

The spiritual energies are forces of healing and life.

The more receptive the soul is for the forces of healing and life, the more the organism receives from the divine principle.

I repeat: If the soul has a lot of spirit power, if it is permeated by light, then the human beings are also mostly healthy and their life positive. This then has an effect on the number and activity of quanta. These people have more spiritual part-powers, more quanta, which are primarily active for them invisibly.

People oriented toward this side of life, whose souls have little life energies, will have to bear their own self-made fate either in this or in later lives, insofar as they do not realize in time why they live as human beings, and then orient their thinking and living to God. In them, the number of spiritual part-powers is low and is effective, that is, visible, predominantly in the material realm.

May this short explanation about the spiritual part-powers, the quanta, serve every person who has some knowledge about the interrelations of the so-called quantum activity.

In general, it is enough for My children to know that the more the spirit power is able to flow into the soul and into the physical body, the healthier and more life-affirming the person becomes or is.

Through the energetic forces, the physical body attains higher vibrations and gains distance from those frequency ranges in which pathogens are found and where negative thought forms try to influence the person.

By leading a morally pure life that is oriented to Me, the eternal Spirit, the soul cleanses itself of the ballast that still lies in it and that possibly stems from a former life or from the present existence on Earth.

If, as a result of the spiritual development of the soul, increased spiritual power flows into both soul and body, then the spiritual part-powers in the person's atomic structure also multiply. At the same time, this results in a greater activity of the entire atomic structure of the human being.

I repeat:

Quanta are, among other things, spiritual bearers of energy for the material atoms and the life force for human beings. They are also the key to health.

The more spirit power flows into a person, the more spiritual part-powers are found in the material atoms.

The spirit power determines the life of a person. The more the spirit power flows into soul and person, the more active are the spiritual and material atoms.

The number of quanta also determines the fate of the human being.

Recognize, O human being: Everything is based on energy. The high sources of energy have a positive influence on all base things. The base forces, all negativity, cause a blockage, a congestion, in the human being and in all material existence.

This blockage in a person, triggered by too little spirit power, leads, in turn, to a multiplicity of wrong reactions.

The soul in the human being came into this world to learn and grow spiritually. Those who grow and mature in the Spirit of God can think clearly. People of the Spirit are not scattered, but are composed in every situation of life. Their thoughts do not wander aimlessly, but are ordered and rest in Me, the Eternal. At the same time, however, they are focused on the matter or the activity at hand.

People with a lot of spirit power are disciplined and concentrated. Whatever they do, they do completely. They look each situation calmly and clearly in the eye, thus averting many dangers that would otherwise befall themselves and their neighbors living in their immediate vicinity. Through the concentrated focus on Me, a blockage in the organism or a stagnation in the life of the person concerned rarely occurs.

Recognize: Like makes the like, in turn, fruitful and thereby fortifies itself: Every feeling, every thought, also every word and every way of acting seeks its like again.

The spiritual part-powers in the material atoms, the quanta, also react to the world of feelings and thoughts of the human beings, likewise to their words and actions.

The spiritual part-powers also influence the body rhythm of a person according to their attitude toward life and their way of life.

In all material life forms, these spiritual bearers of life, the spiritual part-powers, are present in the heavenly bodies and in nature as well. The spiritual forces are at work in all material forms, since they, like everything else, are made up of atoms. Without the spiritual forces, matter could not exist. There would be no material atom, if the spiritual part-powers were not effective.

Be it atoms or molecules, the Spirit is in all things. Without the Spirit, life could not exist, because the Spirit is life.

Those who have come to recognize that God is life and that without God nothing can exist will explore more wisely and in greater depth and will ultimately acquire undreamt-of knowledge. Over the course of time, they will realize that the power of thought can achieve everything, both in and around the person and in all of infinity.

Humankind's technology is merely an aid, because human beings have not yet explored their thoughts and the powers of thought. They research external possibilities and means. They do not, however, open the inner being that holds everything within, of which the person can have only an inkling.

People would not need so-called technology if there were a large number of people of one spirit, that is, of one mind: if they were to first develop the Kingdom of God in themselves, which contains everything soul and person need.

Therefore, it is written: Strive first for the Kingdom of God and everything else will flow toward you.

Through the power of positive thinking, many things—depending on the development of the soul and person, all things—can be accomplished, which is possible only to a limited extent with technology.

Behind the pressure and inclination toward technology is nothing else than the soul's inkling that within it there are unexplored powers that are kept latent by material thinking.

All Being would serve people if they would only acknowledge the existence of the eternal power, the Spirit, and would live according to the eternal laws.

What is created in the world through technology corresponds to the soul's inkling. The flying machines, the airplanes, for instance, are nothing but the expression of the inner being: the soul's deep inkling that it could rise above all spaces, continents and worlds—if it were not tied down by wrong thinking and acting.

The search for the generation of energy also corresponds to the inner inkling of the soul that the inner energy, the spirit power in the soul, can bring forth everything that both soul and person need, for, as I have repeatedly revealed, everything is based on energy.

All cosmic energies are in the soul as essence, which would be activated by positive, lawful thinking and living. Since not only the positive, the lawful, but also the negative, the unlawful, come from within, human beings interpret the inkling of the soul even when they—through misdirection—transform the spiritual down to matter. According to their soul burdens, they do this in line with their possibilities. Both the divine energies and the burdens of the soul, starting from the soul, gain entry into the human organism via the quanta. In this way, the human brain, too, is stimulated.

If only worldly things are stored in the brain cells of human beings, if, for instance, they do research for external sources of energy and invent ingenious technical possibilities for generating energy, they come more and more under the influence of forces that strive to bring about the same and like things in this world.

Thus, whatever lies in human beings, positive and negative, will be manifest in the material world—unless the negativity has been recognized and expiated by human beings in time. Then it will experience the transformation from negative to positive energy in the soul. Then the positive will also become more apparent in the world.

Just as people think and live, to the same extent they influence their environment. They will be controlled by negative forces and will be at their mercy until, for the benefit of all people, they give up everything negative—all that cleaves to the world, the striving for self-affirmation—and selflessly bring what is good into the world.

The soul is in the human body to surrender the negative to the eternal Spirit for transformation, so that soul and person can attain higher spirituality and thus contribute to a positive spiritual life in the world.

The spiritual life also has its effects in the spiritual part-powers, which then are not only more active, but also work in the person in greater numbers, especially in the spheres that are invisible to human beings.

The spiritual part-powers, half spirit, half matter, thus the quanta, are also the fertile forces. Among other things, they contribute to the growth of human beings and, above all, to the growth of the nature kingdoms. They foster the life and the ripening process in all of nature.

If these life energies are in accord with the Earth's magnetic field and magnetic currents, then there is a calm and healthy growth. The life forms of the nature kingdoms are not stricken by disease; the fruits of the fields and forests are healthy and the plants blossom abundantly. And the elemental forces of matter, fire, water, earth and air can thus work together in harmony and achieve a healthy balance in nature.

If the harmony of these forces is disrupted, then the nature kingdoms and also human beings fall ill, since the human being is a nature body.

Harmony and disharmony go out from people.

People's behavior toward the nature king-doms, toward the entire Earth, and lastly, toward infinity, also has an effect on every single person. If a person desecrates the Earth and the nature kingdoms, this interferes with the orderly course of events, with the principles of the law of God. Since in all of infinity, all things are attuned to each other—the large influences the small, and the small influences the large—everything is magnetically interconnected. This brings about a continual exchange and flow of energy.

If this energetic interaction is disrupted, the effect of this is felt where the disruption orig-inated. If a disturbance going out from the Earth affects the entire solar system because the Earth is no longer in harmony with the stars, then this in turn has an effect on and in the Earth: The mating of the animals is disturbed; plants become extinct; other species emerge; stones and minerals attain a corresponding radiation and people oriented to matter also suffer. Everything is in communication with everything else.

For instance, during the time of the full moon, the spiritual part-powers—which are one time spiritual and then again material, depending on their intensity—have an increased effect on the seeds and on all species of plants that blossom, grow, or ripen in each case. If the interaction between the Earth and the stars is disturbed, then also disturbances occur in this regard in and on the Earth and in the human being.

At full moon, the energies of the moon have a stronger influence on the genital organs of men and women, and on the genital organs of *those* animals that have part-souls.

If the forces of both man and woman, and of *those* animals that have part-souls are not in harmony and in harmonious interaction with the radiation of the moon, then deformities at birth or deviant wishful thoughts can be the result, for instance, same-sex activity.

All people are urged to change their ways at every moment. This means that by way of their conscience or impulses from their guardian spirit, they are admonished to shape their life spiritually, to think positively and to become selfless. In this way, the energies in the human being can be harmonized and can then again communicate with the eternal, cosmic, harmonious energies. The communication with the cosmic, harmonious forces then brings about peace, harmony and love in the person and on the Earth.

Those who recognize the divine power in everything that lives and can feel into the life and recognize a part of themselves in the life will shape their life positively and thus approach their neighbors selflessly and recognize their life in all life forms. Those who recognize themselves in nature, since the human being is a nature body, will gradually become friendly, loving and of good will toward their neighbor.

Those who observe nature carefully come to realize that it is a part of themselves.

People can recognize their own life in nature; both the positive, God-pleasing life, as well as the negative, self-centered life. Nature shows them how they should be or how they are.

The spiritually alert person recognizes that life forms a unity. Human beings, animals, plants and stones, even the stars, form a unity. Those who makes friends with nature, the plants and herbs will also be guided, strengthened and re-vitalized again and again by the spiritual forces of nature.

People who are close to nature, that is, people who recognize the ruling hand of the eternal energy, God, in all things will also think, live and act accordingly.

Many plants are medicinal plants.

If possible, one should not use solely dried plants that may have been picked the year before. Instead, those medicinal plants should be used that the present season offers the person, that is, fresh medicinal plants. In fresh plants and herbs, the quanta activity is considerably higher than in dried plants. This is why these fresh medicinal plants or herbs have a much higher vibration than dried ones.

As long as the sap is still in the plant, the effectiveness in the inner life of the plant is stronger than in a dried one. This means that plants that still have sap or are full of sap have a much higher vibration than dried ones. The life force of a fresh plant has a direct effect on the corresponding properties of the plant, and on the organ associated with the plant. A plant filled with sap, freshly picked plants and medicinal herbs are directly irradiated by the cosmic energies. Dried plants and herbs are only indirectly irradiated, namely, by the planetary constellation effective at the time of application.

Plants and herbs can also take on the thoughts of those people who have picked and dried them, or who bought them after they were dried.

Everything is radiation. This is why the critical factor is when and where and with what attitude, the plant was picked.

It also makes a difference whether a plant species grows beside a brook, or in a flowering meadow. It makes a difference whether a plant grows on the wayside or is found in the garden or in a field.

Since everything is based on radiation and radiation varies, a particular plant species can have different properties depending on its location and on the person who picked it.

In the winter months, dried plants and herbs are mostly used for healing purposes. But then, only those herbs should be used that have grown and blossomed in late summer or autumn, because the quanta activity is even stronger in these plants.

As soon as the spirit power flows into matter via the quanta, it becomes a characteristic of the material substance and form, in accordance with the activity of the quanta.

This form is an expression of that part of the spirit power that is visible in the world. The substance is the material, the life for matter, for human beings, animals and plants.

I further reveal that the plants, especially the medicinal plants, resemble human organs in their form. The form of a plant shows a wise person for which organ it was created by the Creator-Spirit.

Via the spiritual part-powers and via the form, the spirit power ensures the suitability of the medicinal plant for both human being and animal.

The suitability and form of the different kinds of plants is also determined by the magnetic fields. The magnetic fields, which help determine the growth of the plants, bear within, as vibration, the characteristics of the plant species. This, in turn, confirms that everything is contained in all things.

The magnetic fields are different in their vibration. This, in turn, is expressed in the vibration of the plant species, as well as in the vibration of human being and animal.

Despite all this, it also matters on which location the plant grows and where the person concerned lives. This is why one and the same plant can have varying properties; one and the same plant species growing near the water contains other substances than does the same plant growing by the wayside. The substances of the plant near the water contain more elements such as iron, phosphorus and potassium. The same plant by the wayside contains other trace elements, such as copper, nickel, silver or even mercury. It all depends on the location of the plant.

Despite these differing trace elements in one and the same plant species, the Spirit gives His energies to each plant equally, according to the spiritual development of the plant species.

I repeat: The quanta and other spiritual part-powers still unexplored by people form the mechanism for the transfer of the spirit power into matter. It is through these spiritual part-powers, the quanta, that the spirit power flows into the material energy carriers.

The spirit power then produces in the human beings, according to their degree of spiritual development, the corresponding activity of the material atoms.

In animals, plants and stones, too, the spirit power is at work, according to their spiritual development.

Because of the free will from God, human beings are able to intervene in the lawful course of the harmonious interaction of forces, thereby disrupting their lawful functions. But they are unable to disturb the Spirit, which is the life. The Spirit remains unaffected by human thinking, feeling and wanting.

For instance, severe mood swings in people may be attributed to the instability of their spiritual consciousness. Such mood swings also have an influence on the activity of the spiritual part-powers, on the quanta. If these tend more toward the material side, that is, if they are more active in the visible sphere, they then temporarily form a barrier and diminish the flow of the spirit power. Among other things, this can then lead to mood swings, which were, however, preceded by negative thoughts, words and actions, that led to the partial blockage of the spirit power.

I repeat: The more spiritual part-powers are active in the material atoms, the healthier people are or the quicker they become healthy.

Therefore, O human being, make the effort to find your way to the higher spheres and the harmonious powers, through a lawful, positive life. In a higher radiation, pathogens will not feel well and will leave your body very quickly.

Regarding the quanta, this means that through a person's positive way of feeling, thinking and acting, the number of quanta increases, through which the radiation of the person becomes more light-filled and broader. The result is health, happiness and contentment. Therefore, become selfless!

Begin the day with Me!
A morning alignment

Human beings are not able to do anything on their own. The earthly body is not viable, unless I, the life, permeate, sustain and vivify it. Therefore, recognize: You are nothing without Me.

For this reason, let go of your arrogance. Arrogance is a barrier to humility. Arrogance scatters, humility unifies.

A humble person who knows about the law of life, that I, the life, Am, will begin the day with Me, the eternal power, the Spirit, and also conclude it with Me, the life.

Humble people are children of light, who not only bring light into dark rooms but also into hardened hearts. They often light up the heart of tired, worry-laden, worldly persons who grumpily go to their workplace.

Therefore, begin the day with Me!

Align yourself daily more with the eternal laws. Meditate about the life behind matter and be aware that I Am the life.

Open yourself to the forces of love by self-lessly loving your fellow people and all forms of life. Then the power of life will flow to you, and you will attain what I have revealed to you: peace, harmony and love. These result in health, happiness and contentment.

Let positive, highly vibrating thoughts and words flow into your inner being already in the early morning. They are light-filled and bright forces that harmonize you and give you a positive orientation for the day that is about to begin. Affirm My power in you with words such as the following:

I am cosmic consciousness, a child of the All, endowed with eternal life.

Continue to speak words into your inner being according to the following:

Life is health.
Life knows neither illness nor worry.
I am healthy and full of vitality.

I affirm the power of the All-Highest
in Christ.
Throughout the day I am concentrated
and oriented to the eternally revealing
life force flowing in me.
My thoughts remain orderly.
I now concentrate on the task that
lies before me.

The forces of the All flow through me,
because I am a child of the All.
In me, the fullness of the Godhead
is effective, the all-prevailing and
maintaining eternal law.
The light permeates me. It frees me.

I am free. I am concentrated and aligned
with the essential.
The forces of the All flow in me.
The almighty power works through me.

The following prayer thoughts may also be prayed into the inner being several times. They keep soul and person fresh and bring about a stabilization of consciousness and a focus on the activity to be carried out during the day:

Heavenly Father,
Your Spirit dwells in Me.
I am your son, your daughter,
eternally living, eternally being,
for You are the life in me.
I am a child of infinity,
a cosmic light-filled being,
because You, the Spirit of infinity,
dwell in me.

Everything that depresses me and wants to influence my concentrated, oriented life,
I place into Your kind hands, trusting and believing in You.

Through Christ, My Redeemer, I want to forgive with all my heart, all those human

beings and souls whom I did not forgive
in former lives.
I also ask for forgiveness of all those people
and beings about whom I have thought or
spoken unjustly or whom I have treated
wrongly in this or in a former life.

I also ask forgiveness for the unlawful
thoughts, words and deeds that keep
coming up in me.
I want to fulfill God's will.

I affirm the Absolute.
I fulfill the Lord's will.
The eternally streaming love stands by me.
I fulfill the love, the law of life.
It will be manifest through me.

I entrust myself to the omnipresent Spirit,
who is the life, who guides the destiny of
infinity and the destiny of all His children.
The Lord wipes out what is not according to
the eternal law of life.

However, what I must bear,
I bear in patience.

May the will of the Lord be done.

Recognize and take My words to heart every day anew: Go out and strive henceforth to sin no more, neither in thoughts, nor in words and deeds.

Then you will be able to achieve everything that is good for you and your neighbor, in your family, at work, and in the world.

Talk little and think even less!
Speak only if it is essential!
Have noble and good feelings.
Refine yourself!

Do your daily duties with equanimity, aligned with the All-harmony, with God. Then you will be protected by the almighty power. This holds true for all people.

These directions should be observed especially by those who bear responsibility for their neighbor. Here, I particularly address the physicians who often manipulate the human body, using it as a test object.

Those who do not recognize themselves do not recognize their neighbor either. However, those who recognize themselves, who have suffered through many things and have found their way to a God-pleasing life will also recognize their neighbor.

Those who recognize themselves will also penetrate to the deep layers of the human ego, recognizing people as they are and not as they pretend to be.

This is especially important for the physician who should support the patient mentally and physically. To find the cause of an illness, the physician should first observe the patient. For every stirring and movement of the body, the entire outer appearance, as well as the direction of the patient's gaze reveal much.

For instance, if the eyes are restless, if the patients cannot look into the physician's eyes, if they look down at the floor or at the wall, then the causes may be the following:

People who look down at the floor hide their difficulties or do not want to let go of the suffering they bear.

Shyness may also be the cause. But even shyness hides a human complex that influences the patient and burdens the subconscious and possibly the organs.

Those who direct their eyes toward the wall are narrow-minded. They are unable or unwilling to accept things, not even physicians and their suggestions and prescriptions.

Those who look out the window want to flee from what exists and is active in them. They don't want to accept either themselves or the physician, nor do they want to hear what the latter has to say.

Those who seriously want to study the patients and their soul to find out the causes of an illness should also pay attention to their way of speaking:

Quick speaking indicates insecurity. The patient wants to hide something that could perhaps give information about the indisposition or even the illness.

Extremely slow speaking indicates lethargy in the person. Such a person has a limited capacity for comprehension. The cause in the body may be a sluggishness of the organs or a slackness of the vessels and intestines.

The shape of the body, too, indicates what is present in the subconscious or in the soul.

Skinny people are often quarrelsome, dominant and jealous. Everything relating to "addiction" should be given special attention with such types of people.

Obese people tend to laziness of the mind; they are the indolent types who look for the causes in their fellow people but seldom in themselves. Obese people often seem to be good-natured, but in many cases this is misleading because of their indolence.

Therefore, it is misleading to speak of obese people as being good-natured. In many cases, the appearance is deceiving. Within, for the most part, they are a volcano. Often they are merely too lazy to let out what they think. But when they literally explode, these types of people turn red with anger and irritation. This indicates a very intense activity of the subconscious.

The red coloring or even the intensified blue of the veins tells the physician not only that the subconscious is boiling over, but also that the condition of the nerves and the composition of the blood, the blood circulation and the vessels should be checked.

The color and shape of the clothes also tell the doctor where to start with the patient to find out where the causes lie.

Every person is a mirror for those who know themselves. Every person is a mirror that tells what they think, how they live and where the causes of the illness or indisposition lie.

People who repress a lot themselves, but think a lot about their neighbors and condemn them are very unforgiving people. Very often their thoughts are in the past. They brood over things long since passed and that can no longer be changed. Nevertheless, they are preoccupied with events that happened long ago. They cannot get over the past because they have not yet forgiven the people who were involved at that time.

In this way, people create thought forms that influence them again and again and harm their weakened organs. The cause is the unwillingness to forgive.

In this way, the subconscious of the person concerned is quite intensely burdened. During the day, the reaction of the subconscious is hardly noticeable. But at night, the subconscious becomes active and starts influencing the organs. During the day, these people can control themselves. They can suppress irritability or outbursts of rage. At night, however, when their will is mostly inactive, the subconscious has a much greater effect on soul and person.

Anxiety dreams, which show themselves in various dream images, rise from the subconscious. They can, however, get mixed with occurrences from former lives that are recorded in the soul garments, for the soul, too, is more active at night than during the day.

Thus, the brain activity comes to rest neither by day nor by night: Such people are hounded day and night. Their nervous system is whipped up. The organs find no rest and wear out accordingly.

The human body is a gift from God for the incarnating soul. For this reason, the human body should not be seen as an object on which to try out one's skills through experimentation.

Human beings are beings from God. They should be seen and treated as such—that is, according to the laws of God and not according to the laws, doctrines and conceptions of this world.

If the majority of people were not listening to world-oriented physicians and intellectual opinion-makers, who leave their fellow people little freedom but impose their acquired knowledge and wisdom on them—thus enslaving many of them and making them dependent on them and on medicines and drugs—light could be brought into the darkness, into the causes of illness and misery.

Often medications are prescribed or patients are advised to undergo an operation, both of which may cause more harm than good. If patients have to suffer often their lifelong because of a physician's wrong decision, the physician concerned seldom feels guilty toward the patient.

From the human perspective, there are so many excuses in this world for those who act unscrupulously. The number of unscrupulous people is considerable. They reinforce and protect each other over and over again, and in many cases, circumvent the worldly law—which often monitors and condemns only the good-natured destitute when they transgress the worldly law.

Such things are possible in this world, but not before the eternal law. After their physical death at the latest, the unscrupulous will have to recognize and endure all that they caused their neighbor. Therefore, may everyone examine themselves first, before "laying hands" on their neighbor.

"Being thrown out of balance" and its consequences

The human body may be compared to a scale: In the center of the body, which we consider as the scale, are the digestive organs and the solar plexus. They see to it that the scale, the human being, is in balance.

If the digestive organ is burdened with too heavy and too rich food, there is an effect on the lower part of the body. More blood than is normally good is drawn from the digestive organs.

396

The lower part of the body becomes heavy and the upper part sluggish; the brain cells become tired.

This unbalanced relationship then affects the solar plexus. The central nervous system becomes tense. The person is irritable and, depending on the person's mentality, the tension results in tiredness or aggression.

Hot spices and spicy drinks also cause the scale, the human being, to get out of balance.

Every disturbance of the scale is registered by the subconscious because every disturbance is an action of thought. The impressions, desires and ideas that have been stored there become more active through this and have a stronger effect on the person.

A tired or aggressive person will start remembering things and occurrences that may have happened way back in the past and were hardly remembered. Because of the disharmony of the scale, of the person, things that were in the process of dissolving or drying out in the subconscious are revived again.

If the person now starts pondering about these memories at length and getting annoyed again, then frustration will again come up just as before. The old and long since past is revived. The active subconscious then begins to exercise an influence on the body and the organs and may possibly even disrupt organs that are functioning well.

In this way, even the composition of the blood can be altered, because the tensed-up nerves secrete so-called neurotoxins into the body and the bloodstream. The body becomes ill. It has been poisoned by toxic thoughts were moved and still move around in the person's mind. In this case, heavy, rich or spicy food and spicy drinks were the trigger.

The body rhythm changed. The organism fell into low vibration. Consequently, the subconscious became active. The person began to think and brood more and more about the past.

Thoughts are powers; they influence the body.

The result was and is indisposition, illness or a blow of fate.

So that the seven basic forces become effective in human beings, they have to first change to a positive life. They have to turn to these forces so that they accomplish in them what they desire: health, happiness, peace and harmony.

Therefore, may everyone begin with themselves first.

Everything pure gives and radiates itself. The impure binds and provides only for itself. What comes of this is egoism, constriction, discord and quarrelling.

Therefore, O human being, be watchful and use every moment! Those who want to teach and lead people take responsibility for them. Thus, people who stand by their neighbor in word and deed bear responsibility before God and their fellow people for what they say and do. Whoever wants to support their neighbor in word and deed should have left behind the influence of the purification spheres of Order and Will.

To the physicians, surgeons and
healing practitioners:
Conversations between physician
and patient—
Establishing a diagnosis together—
Causes in the soul—The body rhythm—
Natural remedies, potencies—
Harmony among physicians
and nursing staff—
Hospital equipment and furnishings—
Changing the milieu by prescription—
A positive clinic atmosphere—
Harmonious music and physical exercises—
The seriously ill—"Houses of Health"—
Life counseling by people of the Spirit

I the revealing Spirit, Christ, want to admonish the physicians and surgeons of this world and give them the following advice:

Above all, try to explore the thoughts of the patients!

Watch their body rhythm before prescribing medications or performing an operation!

The attentive physician can recognize from the patient's outer appearance whether problems, difficulties or complexes, depressions or disharmonies are present. If anything like this exists, the physician should explore with the patient what may lie in the subconscious or as a correspondence in the soul, as far as the patient is able to become aware of these things during a conversation. Only then, should the physician prescribe a medication.

The best medicine physicians can give to their patient are positive, constructive thoughts and words. Coming from a physician, they can dispel many a complex, many a depression or inferiority complex in the patient.

Worry, hardship, disharmony and the like are also resolved if the physicians respond to their patient in the right way.

I appeal to physicians and healing practitioners: Give Me, the Spirit, the opportunity to become more active in the patients, in My human children!

Again, I enjoin all physicians and practitioners: Instruct the patients about the power of positive thinking and about the healing forces in soul and body! At the same time, prescribe natural remedies but only in low potencies, which predominantly relax and support the nervous system.

Therefore, do not immediately resort to strong medications or the scalpel! First explore the subconscious of the patients and the correspondences in their soul, with which they plague and confront themselves in their thoughts and figure out what causes are in their subconscious and in their soul.

The prerequisite, however, is that physicians and practitioners have first examined themselves and have come to know themselves through the power of actualization.

Every human being consists of spirit, soul and body. Those who treat only the body leave cause and effect in the soul. Whatever remains in the soul comes back into the body. When?

The time is determined by the constellation of the planets and by the person involved. If part of the soul burden is in the subconscious and not yet active there, then it is the person who determines when a physical illness will break out. People's world of feelings and thoughts is decisive, but also their behavior in daily life, how much physical energy they waste through uncontrolled speaking or hectic behavior.

Nature gives itself abundantly in many plants and medicinal herbs. They are given to humankind by God, so that human beings may keep their body healthy.

Medicinal herbs administered as tea or homoeopathic potencies are ultimately merely aids or support in the case of illness. They may well have a partial effect on the soul, but they cannot cancel a soul's debt.

On the other hand, high potencies may influence a soul burden and perhaps cause it to flow out earlier than is lawful. This means that soul and body suffer more under this than they are helped. Such action is not lawful.

As long as someone needs medicinal herbs to cure an illness, they should take them. But they should not rely on them exclusively, because the cause of the illness lies in their wrong thinking and living.

Those who consciously absorb the spiritual essences from the medicinal herbs, by virtue of their feelings and thoughts, and shape their life positively, also cause their soul to be filled with life and strength.

However, medicinal herbs cannot take away a soul burden. For this to happen, the person has to contribute their part by living a God-pleasing life.

And avoid thoughts of fear.

Recognize that what does not lie in your soul cannot affect you—unless you act carelessly.

If your soul is purified for the most part, if no dark shadows are in it—which are correspondences and form the magnets for the negativity—then nothing negative can befall you.

It is quite different when you are joined with other people through a spiritual mission. Then the mission has priority and, for you especially, this means that the one carries the burden of the other.

If in you is only lightness and brightness, then you will attract only lightness, brightness and friendliness. Both the pure and the impure in you is a magnet. The pure attracts only the pure, the impure only impureness.

For all those who are seeking, here are some words to remember.

It is not the knowledge of this world that makes a human being wise.

Only the recognition and fulfillment of the spiritual laws enlighten human beings and make them conscious and healthy children of God, truly wise ones.

More words to remember for physicians and healing practitioners:

Those who truly want to help their fellow people should first help themselves by developing the spirit powers that are effective in them, and then putting them to use for the benefit of their neighbor.

Those who have grasped and actualized this will not only prescribe medications for the patient or soothe the organism with drugs. They will explain to those seeking healing that thoughts, words, colors, forms, sounds, light physical exercise and meditation will bring them the desired calm and harmony—and at the same time, they will relax the nervous system with natural remedies and support the body. This holistic therapy is effective for both soul and body.

People who are in the school of the Spirit and live in the actualization of the laws could be of great help to physicians and surgeons.

People of the Spirit see deeper and are often able to recognize what the patients really need and where the physicians should begin their diagnosis, so that those seeking healing may attain relief and healing from their suffering. It is, however, unavoidable that the patients seeking healing cooperate in figuring out and localizing the causes of their indisposition or illness. The diagnosis cannot be established by the physician alone, but by the physician and the patient together.

As soon as the patient's nervous system has calmed down and stabilized, the symptoms, the physical signs and signals can be studied more precisely. Every active body gives indications of where and what it is lacking.

Those who have learned to understand the language of their own body, the language of the organs and cells, are also able to interpret the body language of their neighbor, the language of the organs and cells. With signs and signals, the living organism will itself give an answer as to where the cause of its illness lies and how it might be remedied or what needs to be done to obtain relief and healing.

The body rhythm also gives indications of the body's disorders. Among other things, it is the barometer of soul and body. The physician as well as the healing practitioner can orient themselves to it to make a correct diagnosis.

People's body rhythm indicates whether a lot or little life force flows through them. The sound of the nervous system and of the organs constitutes the body rhythm.

The diversity of species of plants, herbs, flowers, trees and shrubs also have their special rhythm, a cosmic sound that corresponds to their spiritual development.

If the body rhythm of a person seeking healing is not mostly in accord with the rhythm of nature or with a certain medicinal herb, then neither nature nor the herb can work in the ailing organ as well as they could if the rhythms of the human organism and of the healing plant were in consonance.

The whole organism is melody.

Every organ has a special tone. All organs together, including glands and hormones, result in the body's melody. The body rhythm corresponds to the sound of the body.

The sounds of the organs are not perceivable to the human ear or to instruments. The body rhythm, however, is visible and ultimately audible as well. Restless people make a lot of commotion around themselves. Calm people are introspective, making little of their concerns.

Calm people, whose consciousness has been schooled by the actualization of the eternal laws, are attentive, concentrated and receptive. Calm people aligned with God can grasp more in one instant than a noisy person often cannot grasp in several hours or even days and years.

People of the Spirit are also able to grasp and absorb the material and spiritual substances of herbs because they are well-balanced and introspective. This is why they have a harmonious body rhythm that resembles the rhythm of nature.

Those who wants to make use of the cosmic forces that are effective in nature and in all Being must first be willing to change their life and orient themselves to the cosmic forces, to the laws of infinity and to nature. Here, too, holds true: Like attracts like. High powers strengthen and enrich each other. Human energies that have been transformed down, energies of wanting to be, to possess and to have, have a destructive and weakening effect.

The orientation and the goal are decisive. If people are not in the rhythm of nature, if they ignore the laws of nature, natural remedies can be of only little help to them.

If physicians, surgeons and healing practitioners would follow My eternal law, they could truly be servants of the Spirit to humankind.

This world needs spiritually awakened people as naturopaths, who draw on nature and use the herbs of nature to serve and help their neighbor. If physicians, surgeons and healing practitioners were to give more room in their midst to people of the Spirit, then the hospitals would be friendlier, the operating rooms smaller, the rooms for physical exercises and meditation, however, larger. Then there would be Christ-healers in the hospitals, who would lead the people, My children, to their indwelling Christ-power, the inner healing power, and stimulate the spirit power in them to increased activity.

To a greater or lesser extent and according to their consciousness, every person longs for beauty and friendly surroundings; this is determined by the soul. The spirit being, called soul in its burdened state, came from purity and beauty. It has all the harmonious forces of love and wisdom. The divine in the soul reminds the human being of the perfection, of the purity and beauty of heaven. The spirit being came from there and it will return there through Me, the Christ. The souls transmit these impulses to the human beings who then want to build themselves up with all that is harmonious and beautiful. This is why we should not put ourselves under undue pressure, thinking that when we have awakened to spirituality we will have to live in caves or dilapidated houses.

Many people think that someone who has awakened to the inner power, to spirituality, no longer has any need for external things. This is an error. It is said: As within, so without. This does not mean luxury, but rather everything that is beautiful, noble, and natural, that is to say, what is within the realm of possibility.

Those who regard the Earth recognize the abundance and diversity with which the Divine shows itself, with its colors and forms, with its minerals, plants and animals, so that people take delight in them and elevate their soul to ever more beautiful and pure spheres.

People of the Spirit should make their surroundings beautiful and friendly, but not live in luxury and excess.

As people think, so do they live and work. It is similar with their surroundings, too. Harmonious colors, shapes and sounds are vital for a human being. They have a positive effect on both soul and person and fashion their life harmoniously. Many a negative and brooding thought vanishes while looking at a beautiful painting or a beautiful landscape or a harmoniously furnished room.

Harmony is the life of the human body.

If people live in constant disharmony, then they themselves shorten their earthly life.

Through disharmony, the cells in certain areas of the body die off more quickly. As a result, the formation of new cells is not always guaranteed to the necessary extent. This leads to considerable complications in the organism, because the fresh cells then have to perform more. This leads to a weakening of the organs.

Disharmonious vibrations also have an effect on the genes, the genetic make-up, and may activate genetic traits that are not beneficial to the person and that may not have had to be experienced and lived through if the person had lived and acted in a lawful way.

Therefore, all human beings are the architects of their life and the builders of their fate.

Harmony prolongs the life on Earth. Disharmony shortens the earthly life.

Therefore, particularly in clinics or hospitals, great value should be placed on harmonious colors, shapes, sounds and fragrances.

Sick, bedridden people have a lot of time. They perceive their surroundings much more intensely than healthy people who stay in their rooms for only a short time. Sick people in general are much more aware of their surroundings than healthy people. They not only register what is harmonious or dissonant but also absorb it deep in their inner being.

Harmonies which have their expression in colors, shapes, fragrances and sounds are refreshing for the soul. The soul builds itself upon these. That is its life. It is reminded of the eternal homeland. Through this reminder, the soul then releases positive forces such as joy, hope and assurance. They are the best medications for the organism.

The demise of the physical body is already established with the first cry of the newborn child. The human body is granted a certain period of time, depending on the state of the soul and its burden. However, it is the individual persons who decide through their way of thinking and living, whether their physical body passes away prematurely or reaches the limit of its potential age—or whether they even attain the grace to live longer in the temporal, which then possibly excludes a reincarnation for the person. Whatever can be expiated on Earth in the course of years can often be achieved only over a very long cycle of expiation in the spheres beyond time and space.

Therefore, O human being, endeavor to lead a harmonious life. Watch your behavior and react in a lawful way when human thoughts such as hatred, envy, discord, jealousy and thoughts of the past want to shake up your soul and your organism.

Balanced and harmonious people affect their fellow people like the first rays of the spring sun or like several cosmic suns.

Through the balance of those who are oriented to God, the neighbor who encounters such people, who comes together with them, can regain equanimity. Thus, it is always a matter of how you meet your neighbor, not how your neighbor should meet you. Those who seek harmony will also find harmony.

The measure of harmony that you radiate also affects your neighbor. Just as strife and dispute are contagious, so is harmony.

Harmony among the physicians, among the personnel and in the furnishings of hospitals brings about hope, assurance and peace in the soul and body of those seeking healing.

Those who have found harmony will gradually be guided from within. They no longer seek proof. They have the proof in themselves.

Those who radiates harmony from within to without are close to Me, the Eternal.

People of the world whose senses are directed to without are constantly looking for proof. Without proof they can hardly accept anything. For hours on end, they talk and argue about things that ultimately, they cannot understand anyway. In doing this, they waste a lot of life energy. Those who engage in arguments are themselves not convinced of what they argue about with their fellow people.

Truly knowing people are wise. They do not argue, they know. Only unknowing people engage in arguments. Arguments affect the nerve center. They cost a lot of life energy to all those involved.

People who relate only to matter want to impose their opinions on others and have their knowledge recognized. Through such behavior, their organism tenses up more and more, because as soon as people of themselves want something, they commit an act of violence against themselves.

Arguments also create thought structures of incomparable dimensions. Such thought structures then eat away at the nerve center of the persons involved and often prompt a sensitive person with weak nerves to commit acts of violence and other excesses, even acts of immorality.

Excesses and assault, which often occur after a fierce argument, indicate a lack of energy. The person has wasted much life energy through unnecessary talking, through argument. The loss of life energy causes tension. Tension then presses toward discharge, toward relaxation. The person either becomes violent or creates relaxation by excesses of various kinds.

However, those who are thrifty with their life energies will become more sensitive to higher life forces.

The path to spirituality, to the permeability for higher values, results in a balanced, harmonious and selfless life.

As I have already revealed, people who are in a process of transformation from the human and materialistic to higher spirituality will also change in regard to their outer appearance, to their clothing and home.

People of the Spirit dress in an orderly and clean way. The colors of their clothing are harmoniously coordinated. They prefer bright and light fabrics, just as their inner being is bright and light and sunny.

The same thing happens in their apartments and houses. Here, too, many things will change when the person has awakened from the material to the spiritual, when the inner light gradually radiates to without and wants to find its external expression. The apartments and houses of spiritual people become brighter and the furniture more graceful and lighter.

In the same or like way as it is with people in their inner condition, so do they present themselves and their external environment.

Clothing and dwelling reflect the inner being of a person. It is not luxury that is a sign of inner beauty, but the simplicity of clothing and dwelling and their light and bright colors and shapes. Externally, these persons show what their inner state is like.

With this repetition, I want to direct yet another appeal to the physicians.

To shape the life of the patients harmoniously and to achieve deep harmony of soul and body, it is not only the aspect of medications that needs attention. Much more important is the attention given to harmonizing the soul.

The physicians should change their way of thinking and, for instance, recommend that their patients wear light and bright clothing to support the healing process. The colors should be harmoniously coordinated. Also, a change of residence or new furnishings or new wallpaper will change the mood of the patient. A change of surroundings is advisable, too.

Particularly a change of surroundings is often decisive: The new environment evokes a completely different way of thinking in the healthy as well as in the sick person. When people get away from the thought complexes clinging to wallpaper, furniture, clothing and the many different objects that influence and stimulate them accordingly, then a new world will open up to them. Positive thoughts may awaken and bring harmony to soul and body.

The same impressions, the old milieu, constantly affect people and remind them of the past or of events that they can often overcome only through a change of milieu—or through a complete transformation of their old habits.

A change in external circumstances is often more beneficial than any medication, or it improves the effect of medications or natural remedies.

Humankind should also be instructed about the effect of fragrances, especially the physicians, so that they can treat their patient with this approach, too.

Through heavy fragrances, an already existing sentimentality may cause a person to become weary of life.

Fragrances can be perceived by soul and person. Among other things, they might disturb or even harm the nervous system. Therefore, artificial fragrances should be used only under specific conditions and in a small dose.

Recognize that a healthy and light-filled soul also emits a pleasant whiff from the inner life, the fragrance from the pure Being, because the soul has become light-filled and bright.

Hence, one can also draw conclusions about the state of the soul from body odor.

If people learn to think lawfully, they will also live lawfully.

Life as a whole is melody and fragrance. Soul and person smell according to their way of thinking and living.

All these indications are instructions for life to stay or become healthy. They also apply to physicians who bear great responsibility for the good or the woe of their patients.

If hospitals were designed and furnished in a more friendly way and did not convey only the impression of illness, suffering and lingering illness, there would be more joyful, positively minded people in these buildings as well. They would be houses for inner recognition and inner edification. In this way, the patients would find a positive attitude toward their illness and be able to accept and bear many things.

In the clinics of this world, everyone speaks only of illness and suffering. Through this, an atmosphere of vibrations of illness, fear and worry develops. These vibrations cling to objects, to beds, chairs, closets and instruments. All the rooms, including the operating room, are contaminated with them. The building and the surroundings radiate whatever happens within the rooms in thoughts, words and deeds.

422

The fear of death, too, attracts danger. The fear of death can cause the surgeon to become nervous and make wrong decisions or mistakes during the operation, which can then lead to death.

In a clinic, no constructive, positive force can be developed as long as physicians and nurses do not have a radiation of energy that is constructive and motivating and as long as the patients are mere objects to them—or even prisoners of their ideas, instructions and habits.

Where there is no sense of community between physician and patients, there can be no inner communication. The objects, the human beings, say "yes" to the authority, the physician, while, at the same time they are filled with fear and worry and secretly build up thoughts of their possible demise.

For many, so-called death is something shrouded in mystery because only few people have lived rightfully and have asked themselves about the meaning of life. During their life, only few think about the process of passing away, about where they come from and where they are going. Those who have seriously dealt with these questions, by living day by day in such a way that they can pass on at any time, will also—in the moments of a critical situation, such as illness—sensitize their soul and their whole body in such a way that the physician is favorably inspired and makes the right decision. Therefore, in many cases it depends on both the physician and the patient whether an illness ends with physical death or with a continuing life on Earth.

If only suffering, fear, lingering illness and fear of death emanate from clinics and hospitals, no positive force can enter there—and therefore cannot be effective either.

Hospitals and clinics, in particular, should radiate a positive atmosphere that has a calming, constructive and strengthening influence on those who seek healing. However, since many clinics and hospitals lack spiritually knowledgeable doctors, aids and nurses, such houses are often places of horror.

If physicians and staff were to think, live and act in a spiritual way, then in many cases natural remedies would be sufficient to stimulate the body to self-healing through the Spirit. Thus, in many cases, a surgical intervention in the organism, an operation, could be avoided.

Once again, I want to draw attention to the physical exercises about which I have already revealed: An excellent contribution to health comes from harmonious physical exercises with accompanying harmonious music.

Harmonious music combined with body exercises and above all positive thinking call upon the cell tissues to accept more life forces, to activate themselves and to stabilize the body. Thereby, also the quanta in the atomic structure of a person are stimulated and cause, which was already revealed, that the person receives more spirit power through Me, the Inner Physician and Healer.

The harmonious, lawful influence on soul and person brings about a higher vibration of the cells and muscles. In the physical body, it also causes the normalization and stabilization of the circulation. In this way, both soul and body attain a raised body rhythm, a higher vibration.

If soul and body are in harmony, then the human being is also receptive to the spiritual life counseling and to the spiritual healing and life forces.

If through these simple methods, both soul and body are prepared for the higher life forces, for the spirit powers in the human being, then, in many cases, human beings would gain a positive attitude toward their illness and their environment.

With these simple aids, a despondent person may attain mental and physical balance and gain harmony with the environment. Thoughts of illness and suffering are then replaced by confidence, hope, thankfulness and the will to be completely healthy again. This is the proper motivation for the cell structure, for the cell state, which is then activated through My eternal power and is ready to receive My healing currents.

Many hospitals also lack explanatory lectures on the power of positive thinking as well as related literature.

The power of thought is manifold. Those who know how to apply their thoughts in the right way become creative, sensitive, healthy and happy.

As already revealed, positive, high and noble thoughts are the best medicine. If the body were prepared with appropriate harmonious music and purposeful physical exercises, many a patient could be spared much.

The physical body is a "body of motion" and as therapy also requires movement in fresh air or in harmoniously furnished rooms; because colors, forms and sounds have a combined effect on the soul and the person.

Special attention and care should be given to the seriously ill. Many people suffer greatly under the burden of a soul debt that is affecting their body. They, in particular, need special devotion and care.

If a soul burden flows out, not only the person, the body, suffers, but also the weakened soul, which is low in energy during this time. The more selfless devotion the person receives from their neighbor and the more a beloved person participates in the life of the patient, the more meaningful the life of the person seeking help and healing becomes again. The suffering soul, too, gratefully accepts this selfless service.

The staff at the clinics as well as the members of the family concerned are advised to integrate the seriously ill person in their daily routine. It would be good to give the ill, even the seriously ill, minor or major tasks, depending on the intensity of their physical suffering. In this way, they sense that they are still needed.

Even the seriously ill should participate in the uplifting forces that result from harmonizing music and harmonious physical exercises. If the seriously ill are bedridden, they nevertheless can be taken to pleasant rooms set up for music and exercise, which should also serve as rooms for meditation. In this way, the bedridden patients can participate in the physical exercises of their fellow patients. Their senses of sight and hearing register the movements and the harmonious sounds. The muscles and the cells, the person's whole organism, gratefully absorb the harmonious sounds and they automatically react to these sounds, which trigger vibrations in muscles and cells. These harmonious vibrations are an inner massage, as it were; the nerves and organs relax and the positive forces are activated within the person: Hope, confidence and thoughts of wholeness may result.

Even a soul poor in energy thankfully accepts the vibrations of the harmonious sounds and the movements of the body, or even just the vibration of the muscles. The vibrations of the music and the movements of their fellow patients cause the atomic structure of the soul and body of the seriously ill person to attain a higher vibration. This also brings about a mental-physical balance in the patient.

In many clinics the seriously ill drowse and vegetate. They are given pain-killing and sedative medications. Such people are often nothing but experimental objects for those who regard the physical body as an essential factor, but know little or nothing about the soul, which registers everything. It is they who often inflict unimaginable agonies on the spirit body, the soul.

All doctors and relevant specialists should be advised once again to pay more attention to the bearer of life energy, the soul. If the soul regains health, then the body will also become healthy. If the soul is healthy, then the body is also healthy.

Once again I appeal to all physicians:

See the patient as a part of you! Whatever you do not want others to do to you, do not do to your neighbor.

Thoughts are undreamt-of forces.

Positive, harmonious forces uplift the emotional life and promote the power of recovery.

Positive forces give comfort to the hopeless. They give courage to those who suffer. They give

430

strength to the joyless, so that they may be glad again.

Love your fellow people and help them, and you will be loved in return; for everything that goes out from you that is selfless, good and beautiful, you will receive again in manifold ways.

Therefore, let the hospitals become houses of health. Then the world will brighten and people will come together in thankfulness and joy toward God, the life, the healing power.

When convalescent patients return to their environment, to their family and their place of work and are then confronted with their old habits and problems, they cannot always keep their distance from them. Then the danger of a relapse looms. In these situations, the recovering persons should have a counselor to support them, with whom they can talk about the difficulties that are now arising again.

Verily, I say to all of you, the physicians, the scientists, the theologians, the assistant staff and the sick: Those who apply the methods given by the Spirit in the right way will not only achieve great success, but will also be of great service to humanity.

People in Me, the Spirit, can do great things for suffering humanity.

The world needs Christ and people who think and live in a truly Christian way.

The law on the level of Order says: Ask and you shall be given! Seek, and you shall find! Knock, and the door will be opened! This applies to all people—to physicians, scientists, theologians—as well as to all those seeking healing.

So that people find peace, tranquility and help on the path to inner peace, it is necessary to have knowledgeable and spiritual people who know the laws of life from their own experience and not just from books and lectures. People are needed who help and serve from within, totally according to the laws of life. Those who can draw from a wealth of self-experience, who have experienced the holy laws in and on themselves through their actualization are true servants and helpers of humanity.

Ask, and you shall be given! Seek, and you shall find!

There are some people who have come to know the laws of life not only from books, who have not only book knowledge, but who stand in the midst of the fulfillment of the law. It is they who can help the physicians, the theologians and the scientists so that the world may become more light-filled—as well as the hospitals.

In this time of great change, in which cosmic forces are flowing into this side of life more intensely, I, the eternal Spirit, Christ, offer My service again. Those who knock will receive.

May those who want to help their neighbor out of true selflessness work together with Me, the Christ, and with all those who follow Me, with people who fulfill the laws of love and of peace. Happy are those who can grasp this in this time of cosmic change! May those who have ears, hear!

May those who have a heart for their fellow people open it wide to serve their neighbor selflessly!

Intellectual knowledge blinds people to the truth. May those who want to find the truth and draw from the truth act selflessly, without asking what their profit might be, or whether they can acquire prestige, money or possessions for themselves.

O human being, be diligent in the Spirit! Then you can truly change and improve the world, for I want to be with you.

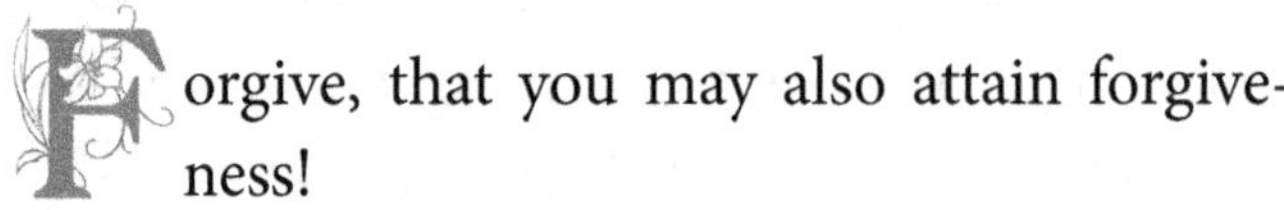

Forgive, that you may also attain forgiveness!

God can forgive you only when you ask for forgiveness and your neighbor has forgiven you. Not just the knowledge of this principle of law is of importance; only the knowledge and its actualization will bring freedom to your soul and to your thoughts. The one who does not forgive or attain forgiveness cannot return to the Father's house.

If you ask for forgiveness and your neighbor does not forgive you, you cannot attain perfection either. Therefore, pay attention to your thoughts, words and deeds. Every thought, every word and also every action sets you free or ties you to what you condemn or want to keep, be it people or objects.

Therefore, O human being, watch your thoughts, words and deeds. They can be your undoing or your well-being. If the world had recognized, grasped and actualized the meaning of this phrase "forgive, so that you, too, may be forgiven," humanity would not be on the precipice of intolerance, ignorance and destruction.

My explanations clarify the law of cause and effect and thus the teaching of reincarnation as well.

The soul of people who do not repent, who neither ask for forgiveness nor forgive, who keep on judging, condemning and harming their neighbor in manifold ways will return again in accordance with the law of cause and effect, of sowing and reaping.

The links in earthly life that lead to further burdens are manifold. Often insignificant negative thoughts are reinforced by other similar thoughts, so that a negative field of thought develops, which I also call a correspondence. This field of thought called a thought complex or correspondence is taken up by the magnetic soul and forms in the soul particles—by changing the five spiritual atomic types—the soul debt. The thought complex, the correspondence, then overlays the soul's core of being, which— the more correspondences, the more soul-debt complexes are present—decreases its intensity, the radiant power.

The manifold causes which lead to a soul burden, to a thought complex that is absorbed by the magnetic soul, can never be explained in detail with words. The law of cause and effect is the law of karma; it is the justice of God. Only sensitive people who are oriented to God feel and

436

know the significance of the law of sowing and reaping. They grasp it in their souls.

Often an insignificant, negative thought can be the cause of a blow of fate that accompanies and influences people during their whole life long and, beyond that, the soul in the spheres of purification. If such an insignificant thought is reinforced by the same or like thoughts, then a thought complex develops that can have an effect on the disposition and body functions of a person. Then, a single, negative thought can be the target for further negativities, possibly stimulated by external energy fields or by souls. Just as negative thoughts can be intensified by negative forces, in the same way, noble and pure thoughts are irradiated by high powers, by spirit beings, and by the eternal power, God.

Those who sow good, noble thoughts and words and do good in their life create high ideals and values for their future. If, in addition, they have learned to accept everything thankfully, be it joy or suffering, they truly purify their soul and prepare it for the eternal homeland.

Nothing happens by chance, neither in the fine-material spheres nor in matter. Everything is well ordered by the Creator-God. Thus, whatever people sow in their feelings, thoughts, words and deeds, they will reap. This is based on the law of cause and effect.

God is a God of order, even if the worldly person does not want to perceive or to accept the cosmic correlations and connections.

The way back to the Father's house is the path of actualization:

A person cannot find the origin of the wellspring merely by hearing the word. Hearing and reading the word of God, whether from the Bible or from spiritual sources that flow unadulterated from the truth, does not purify the soul or restore it to the image of the Father. Only the law that is lived, the truth that is lived, makes a person free.

Those who expand their consciousness and have raised it beyond the four purification planes will no longer ask, seek or knock; they have found it: The fullness of God is revealed to them.

Therefore, O human being, live in the now. The law knows neither yesterday nor tomorrow. Everything is fulfilled in the now, because there is solely the present. God is not transient. God is eternal. God is the life. Whether you are in the spirit or in the flesh, everything is life.

Become free of yourself! Forgive! Let go of what preoccupies you! Raise your thinking, feeling and wanting to God! And fulfill what is His will. Then your soul will rise, and you will behold, in yourself, the truth that has set you free.

Know that your heart is where your treasure lies. One day, your soul will be there.

The soul of a formerly successful business-man who acquired a lot of money and property, who adorned himself with it and bragged about it and considered his success and his posses-sions his own achievement will be back as a soul to where his heart hung and hangs.

A wife and mother who not only felt very attached to her family, but had bound herself to the members of her family and considered her small parcel as her own, will be back as a soul to where her heart hung.

Two people, for example, have acquired land together and later come into difficulties. They fight fiercely because each one insists on their rights. If no reconciliation is reached before either soul of the quarreling parties leaves its physical body, after its disembodiment it will find itself again where its whole heart, its every thought and aspiration was. As a soul, it may even go on arguing there, continuing to work just as it did before in its earthly garment. It may possibly live for a long time in this pseudo reality until it awakens from its thought pattern.

I have taken but a few drops from the ocean of karmic interrelationships and revealed them briefly.

People of the Spirit do not look back into the past fearfully, nor do they anxiously try to secure their future. They live in the present and realize what possibilities are now offered to them by Me, the Christ.

To be able to atone now, in this present life, for many things, to disentangle the karmic tree of life in this way and to put one's inner being in order, right planning is needed. People of the Spirit plan, but they do not force themselves or their neighbor to carry out what only the law can do anyway. People who live a life of actualization may be sure that the law of love is being fulfilled in and around them. They can let go and plan for the future in accordance with the law.

The opinion of the human being forms the bond which, after the passing of the body, draws the soul back to where it once enjoyed its passions and pleasures as a human being:

If you remain an alcoholic until the end of your life on Earth, your soul will be among alcoholics again. The soul of a glutton will feel at home where there is an abundance of food and stimulants. It will be drawn to where people focus their main attention on pleasures and the like.

The soul of a drug addict will once again be where the same people live, where these substances can be obtained. The one who indulges in desires and passions will once again as soul be among those who think and live similarly.

The soul of a murderer will once again be at the scene of the crime, where the still unatoned vibrations of suffering and pain of his victim adhere and radiate.

The soul of a person who once chose suicide will continue to live and work in the same place as before as a human being. This will be until the time when the body would have reached its physical death according to the law of cause and effect.

God, the eternal law of love, sends unceasingly, giving both soul and human being impulses to awaken and align with His holy consciousness.

Happy are those who have oriented themselves to the highest transmitter, to God! They can be admonished and reminded by Him, and they will realize that it is their loving Father who admonishes His child to change its ways and turn within.

The revelation I have given is showing the way for all people who are of good will.

What has been revealed will be recognized, affirmed and put into practice by a soul that is alert and mature.

My word is not binding—but informs, admonishes and guides.

Those who want to recognize and experience the truth, the law of life in themselves as truth, must first find the way to the truth.

May what I have revealed to My human children give deep insights into the prevailing eternal law, which can be perceived and understood in detail only by those people who have found their way to the truth, who do not confine themselves to the mere perception of words, but who grasp their meaning.

One's own experience of all things can find fulfillment only in a genuine and deep inner vision—not in the word. Words are mere symbols. Those who are unable to look behind the mirror of the words, into the symbolism of the word, will always ask whether what I have revealed corresponds to the truth. They will not recognize the great correlations since they do not know themselves.

The truth lies in you, O human being. The word is merely a guide.

Recognize this and find the way to inner truth. Then you will find Me, your Redeemer, the Inspirer of the eternal truth, for I Am the way, the truth and the life.

Those who have become the truth will hear My voice.

I Am the truth in all Being.

I consciously live through those who live in Me. They have become one with Me. They draw from the fullness and behold the fullness as conscious sons and conscious daughters of heaven.

Amen

Recommended Reading

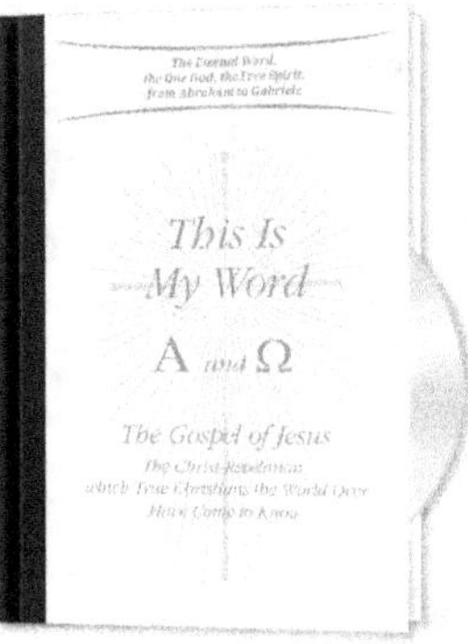

This Is My Word
A and Ω

The Gospel of Jesus

The Christ-Revelation,
which True Christians the World Over
Have Come to Know

Jesus of Nazareth founded no religion. He installed no priests and taught no dogmas, rites or cults. 2000 years ago, He brought the truth from the Kingdom of God: the teachings of the love for God and neighbor toward people, nature and animals, the teaching of freedom, of peace and of unity. He spoke about the God of love, of the Free Spirit—God in us.

In the mighty work of revelation, "This Is My Word – Alpha and Omega," Christ speaks from the Kingdom of God through Gabriele, the prophetess and emissary of God, about the past, the present and the future.

In His work, which is a historic work, He directs Himself to all people, to explain what He as Jesus of Nazareth taught, how His life on Earth took its course, and He shows the correlations in the great work of Redemption that has its origin in the Kingdom of God.

An Audio-CD is included in the book with
The eternal word from the Kingdom of God:
"The Call of the Christ of God" and *"The Appearance,"*
Given through Gabriele, the prophetess of God in our time
1078 pp., HB, Order No. S 007en, ISBN 978-3-96446-313-5
Also available as an E-book

www.ingramcontent.com/pod-product-compliance
Lightning Source LLC
La Vergne TN
LVHW011000200726
843509LV00011B/931